CONGENITAL ANOMALIES – CASE STUDIES AND MECHANISMS

Edited by **Alastair Sutcliffe**

Congenital Anomalies – Case Studies and Mechanisms
Edited by Alastair Sutcliffe

Published by InTech
Janeza Trdine 9, 51000 Rijeka, Croatia

Publishing Process Manager Ana Skalamera

Technical Editor Teodora Smiljanic

Cover Designer InTech Design Team

Additional hard copies can be obtained from orders@intechopen.com

Congenital Anomalies – Case Studies and Mechanisms, Edited by Alastair Sutcliffe
p. cm.
ISBN 978-953-51-0075-1

For EU product safety concerns:
IN TECH d.o.o., Prolaz Marije Krucifikse Kozulić 3, 51000 Rijeka, Croatia,
info@intechopen.com or visit our website at intechopen.com.

Meet the editor

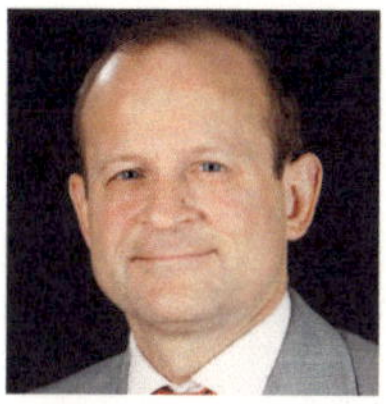

Professor Sutcliffe has been looking after sick children for over 20 years and is fully aware of the potentially devastating effects of congenital anomalies on the health of children and the burden they can put on their parents and health services.

He qualified from the University of Manchester and has spent the last 15 years in academic posts in University College London. As an internationally regarded expert on the health of children conceived from assisted reproductive technologies , since his first seminal studies of children born afer embryo freeze thawing, he has watched the proportion of IVF births rise from 0.5% to the present 2% in the UK, with some coutries double that. Some of his studies have focussed on congenital anomalies. Professor Sutcliffe also has expertise in paediatric therapeutics and is presently conducting studies looking at pharmacovigillance of medicines given to both Mothers in pregnancy and children. Dr Sutcliffe has two doctorates and has received international prizes for his work.

Contents

Preface

Congenital Anomalies – Case Studies and Mechanisms
An introductory text for the student

Chapter 1
- *Hox* Genes and Teratogenic Factors

Within this state of the art book is a series of exemplary chapters which illustrate the shear complexity of understanding of factors which need to be anticipated when considering, mechanisms, aetiology, investigation, epidemiology, and other considerations in human malformations.

Starting with a Chapter 1 on Hox genes and their importance in teratology, the reader is given an in depth understanding as to how these now well understood basic building block control genes are intimately involved in potential structural malformations. Introducing the reader to the idea that genetic errors from simple deletions, missense and other mutations in Hox can have profound implications for the human being in development. From this the student is encouraged to read further regarding potential other genetic bases for malformations and how subtle these changes can be in the fully formed individual. They are reminded and indeed this is a recurrent theme of this excellent 'sampler' book of what a fascinating but highly complicated area of medical science this is.

Chapter 2
- Signalling Mechanisms Underlying Congenital Malformation: The Gatekeepers, Glypicans

Moving to another key concept in malformation aetiology…glypicans I immensely enjoyed this erudite chapter (2) written by one of the world's experts on this topic. The title for the non-expert is quite scary! But enjoy the chapter is it is an excellent example of a way to illustrate a theoretically complex concept 'signalling' via our old friends the glypicans and their key role as gatekeepers of the 'fort.' The reader is encouraged via this exemplary chapter to consider how complex malformations may develop from simple problems at the embryological level.

Chapter 3
- Central nervous system vascular malformations

This Chapter logically leads the student to a broader understanding of how gene malfunction, signalling and other mechanisms start to broaden into gross anatomical malformations and the human being then becomes diseased being. An understanding of the body needs to focus on individual parts which can be affected. In terms of sheer complexity the order of body systems is in order the central nervous system, then the heart and cardio vascular system, then the genito urinary system and so forth.

So it unsurprising that due to its sheer complexity the CNS is most prone to malformations. This is both challenging and has profound implications for the patient. Thus again in this demonstration chapter one is drawn to the malformations as erudite examples of the theme that underpinning complex mechanisms result in gross anatomical problems.

Chapter 4
- Ultrasound Diagnosis of Congenital Brain Anomalies

Continuing the CNS theme here is the only truly clinical chapter in this book. Day to day millions of ultrasound investigations are done worldwide. A major area of their usage is in clinical medicine. When the patient is suspected of a congenital malformation which can present at any age, they present to doctor and are then investigated. Advances in ultrasound scanning which have occurred in my 25 years in clinical practice are used in the diagnoses of anomalies of the CNS more and more especially in the neonate. Herein the student in science of teratology is brought as it were to the bedside with a practical example of how the patient is investigated at the bedside.

Chapter 5
- An Autopsy Case of Congenital Pulmonary Lymphangiectasis Masquerading as Pulmonary Interstitial Emphysema

It is said that most patients who end up in the morgue are found to have incorrect in vivo diagnoses. The historical approach to determining cause of death was via morbid anatomy. In this short chapter this principle is beautifully exemplified with a case incorrectly diagnosed in vivo in which the irreplaceable skill of the gross pathologist, histologist and related are demonstrated reminding the student of the multiple skills and levels of understanding needed to become a malformation expert.

Chapter 6
- Assisted Reproductive Technology and Congenital Malformations

If you are looking up in the sky and you see some white lines which are clearly not clouds, you generally would conclude that these are vapour trails from a passenger jet which has passed by recently. Even if you had not seen the airplane.Welcome to the concept of epidemiology. Possible causation of disease are imputed by evidence that an event has happened. Most individual congenital anomalies are fortunately rare. The only way one can potentially become aware of that risk factor for them is through epidemiological studies using decent datasets with minimal missing data. In this chapter a discussion surrounds the up to 4% of human beings now being conceived with extra help via assisted conception and their much talked about increased risk of birth defects. The senior author is the world's most expert person in this field and the authors' expertise is reflected in the thorough description of studies of congential anomalies after ART and their potential risks according to types of ART (assisted reproductive technologies). This is a final chapter in this introduction to concepts in congenital anomalies.

Enjoy this brief taster in what is a fascinating field.

Professor Alastair Sutcliffe
Institute of Child Health, University College London,
United Kingdom

1

Hox Genes and Teratogenic Factors

Takuya Kojima and Naoki Takahashi
*Department of Applied Biological Chemistry,
Graduated School of Agricultural and Life Sciences,
University of Tokyo,
Japan*

1. Introduction

Exposure to a variety of chemicals is a hazard of daily life. Some of these chemicals have teratogenic potency and may lead to social problems. As an example, thalidomide was prescribed as a sedative and for morning sickness in the late 1950s and caused serious embryonic effects worldwide. To avoid these problems, the development of efficient techniques for the detection of teratogenic substances contained in various chemical compounds is desired. Detection of teratogenic effects using various experimental animals is only partially effective because different phenotypes occur among species. Therefore, effective methods for the detection of teratogenic factors must be based on their molecular mechanisms. However, knowledge of the molecular mechanisms that lead to the different phenotypes caused by teratogenic factors is limited, and useful molecular markers for these factors are not known.

Approximately 30,000 genes in higher organisms are expressed under strict control. This regulation of expression is mainly dependent on transcription factor networks. In higher organisms, there are about five hundred transcription factors that contain a DNA-binding domain and cooperate in the regulation of the expression of downstream genes. Alterations in these regulatory mechanisms result in a variety of problems. In the case of teratogenic factors, abnormal morphogenesis is one of the common findings in exposed embryos. Developmental abnormalities including skeletal malformations, cleft palates, neural tube defects, and cardiovascular anomalies have been found to have a similar causative mechanism, which was revealed in loss- or gain-of-function studies of the transcription factors involved in morphogenesis. The information from genetic analyses is important for the understanding of the molecular mechanism of teratogenic effects.

The present chapter discusses the transcription factors involved in morphogenesis (*Hox*, T-box family, and other homeo-box genes) and the deleterious agents that lead to congenital malformations, and the link between them is explored. We also present recent findings from our group and provide guidelines for the prevention of the risks associated with environmental contaminants. In addition, we speculate on the molecular mechanisms of congenital malformation.

2. Transcription factors for development

The individual cells that make up multi cellular organisms acquire a wide variety of positional information cues from body axes. This local information leads to the formation of tissues and organs and is essential for the maintenance of homeostasis. There are three fundamental axes in multi cellular organisms: anterior-posterior, dorso-ventral, and proximal-distal. Abnormalities in body axis formation caused by genetic or external factors can lead to the development of lesions. Certain transcription factors play critical roles in body axis patterning, along with a wide variety of diffusible factors such as growth factors, BMPs, sonic hedgehog.

In this section, we refer to several transcription factors involved in body axis formation.

2.1 *Hox* genes

2.1.1 Overview of *Hox* genes

Hox genes encode transcription factors that play important roles in the process of morphogenesis along the anterior-posterior axis of the body. In the early 1900s, Morgan and Bridges found abnormal body plan mutants such as the replacement of antennae with legs in *Drosophila melanogaster*. These morphological abnormalities may have been caused by alterations in the expression of genes that contain a characteristic sequence (homeo-box), which were described in 1970. The homeo-box sequence encodes 61 amino acids designated as the homeo-domain and composed of a helix-turn-helix. Through the activity of this homeo-domain, Hox proteins bind a core consensus sequence (5′-TAAT-3′) in target genes and function as transcriptional activators or repressors. In the regulation of the expression of various downstream genes, Hox proteins function as monomers, homodimers, heterodimers, or heterotrimers with cofactors such as Meis or Pbx family proteins (Moens and Selleri, 2006). *Hox* genes are highly conserved across species. In the nematode *Caenorhabditis elegans*, there are seven *Hox* genes in chromosome III that are distributed in intervals of 3.9 Mb. In the fly *Droshophila melanogaster*, eight *Hox* genes are clustered in chromosome 3R, which is referred to as the homeotic complex (HOM-C), and they are located across long interval regions consisting of 9.5 Mb. *Hox* genes are also clustered between 100 kb regions in the mammalian genome but this cluster is tandem duplicated; there are four clusters in the mouse (chromosomes 7, 17, 12, and 2) and humans (chromosomes 6, 11, 15, and 2). These separate clusters are termed Hox A, B, C, and D, respectively.

In normal vertebrate development, there are three important features of *Hox* gene expression. First, the genomic locations reflect the expression in the A-P axis. Generally, 3′ genes are expressed in anterior tissues and 5′ genes in posterior tissues. This phenomenon is termed "spatial colinearity". Second, 5′ located *Hox* genes will have a dominant phenotype to more 3′ located *Hox* genes. This is referred to as "posterior prevalence". The third feature is "temporal colinearity"; 3′ located *Hox* genes in the cluster are expressed earlier than 5′ located *Hox* genes (Mallo et al., 2010). These properties are under strict expressional control; actually a wide range of factors are involved in the control of *Hox* gene expression. A common mechanism of regulation of *Hox* expression is epigenetic control. In general, the silencing of genes is mediated by histone modifications such as the methylation of the promoter region. Polycomb and trithorax group proteins are important modulators of histone trimethylation. The polycomb group and trithorax complexes trimethylate lysine 27 of histone H3 (H3K27) and lysine 4 of histone H3 (H3K4), respectively (Mendenhall and Bernstein, 2008). These histone modifications can be reflected in gene expression states such as inactive in H3K27m3 or active in H3K4m3. In undifferentiated pluripotent cells, two modifications are found in some local regions and are described as a bivalent chromatin domain (Bernstein et al., 2006). These chromatin modifications lead to changes in the accessibility of trans-acting factors that bind to cis-elements. The expression of *Hox* genes is regulated by a wide variety of trans-acting factors: Hox (self-, palalogus-, and another family gene) and other types of transcription factors (Cdx, Rar/Rxr, etc: see below).

Second, small or large RNAs that are independent of protein synthesis regulate *Hox* gene expression. In the *Hox* cluster, there are three miRNA families, namely mir-10, mir-196, and mir-615. These miRNAs are conserved between the fly and humans. Generally, miRNAs have been thought to influence the target mRNA stability and translation. In mammalians, at least 30 of the 39 *Hox* 3′ UTRs have one or more conserved matches to miRNAs like mir-196. The expression of these mir-10 and mir-196 families is complementary to *Hox* gene expression (Mansfield et al., 2004) and is closely linked to posterior prevalence (Hornstein et al., 2005; Yekta et al., 2004). The number of registered miRNAs has recently reached more than 16,000 (miRBase, release 17), suggesting that other miRNAs from outside the *Hox* cluster may contribute to the regulation of *Hox* gene expression. LncRNAs (long noncoding RNAs), which range from several hundred bases to dozens of kilobases, are another type of RNA polymerase II transcribed RNA with a different function from a template for protein synthesis. *Xist*, known as a regulator of parental-specific expression of imprinting genes, is cited as one example (Augui et al., 2011). There are two lncRNAs transcribed from both sides of the *HoxA* cluster. *Hottip*, transcribed from the 5′ site of *HoxA13*, and *Hotairm1*, transcribed from between *HoxA1* and *HoxA2*, are the recently reported lncRNAs that lead to conformational changes in chromatin together with the transcribed *Hox* gene RNA (Rinn et al., 2007; Wang et al., 2011).

The regulation of the expression of the *Hox* cluster genes occurs through a wide variety of mechanisms, and irregularities in this regulation can result in several abnormalities as described in the following sections.

2.1.2 Phenotypes of *Hox* mutants

Loss or gain of function *Hox* mutants show homeotic transformations across species. The identity of body segments is determined by specific combinations of *Hox* gene expression known as the "Hox-code". Alterations in the Hox-code result in abnormalities in morphogenesis along the longitudinal (A-P) axis of the body, termed homeotic transformation. For example, loss of function of the *labial* gene in the fly, which is located in the 3′ region of the cluster, results in the disorganization of cranial structure, which is seen in the formation of the salivary glands. The *antennapedia* mutant is characterized by the replacement of antennae by legs (Hughes and Kaufman, 2002). The HOM-C complex is formed by two gene clusters, the *antennapedia* complex (*ANT-C*) and the *bithorax* complex (*BX-C*). These two complexes are encoded in the same chromosome but are separated by 9.5 Mb. Genetic analyses have shown that *ANT-C* determines the specificity of the anterior thoracic and head regions, and *BX-C* determines the posterior thoracic segments and the abdomen.

In higher organisms, there are 39 known *Hox* genes and the analysis of their function has become increasingly more complex. The analysis of the function of mammalian *Hox* genes in vivo has been carried out through the generation of a large number of *Hox* gene knockout or knock-in mice. These mice frequently show skeletal abnormalities such as alterations in the number of thoracic segments. These phenotypes are explained as resulting from aberrances in the Hox-code (Wellik, 2009). Dramatic phenotypes, such as the replacement of antennae by legs in the fly mutant, are not observed in single gene mutants in mammals possibly because of compensatory effects between the 39 *Hox* genes, especially among paralogous genes.

Individual *Hox* genes have specific functions in various organs. Among skeletal abnormalities, cleft palate phenotypes have been detected in *Hoxa2*$^{-/-}$ mice (Gendron-Maguire et al., 1993). These phenotypes have also been observed in *Hoxa7* and *Hoxb7* gain of function mice (Balling et al., 1989; McLain et al., 1992).

The expression of *Hox* genes belonging to paralog groups 9 to 13 are coordinately detected during limb bud development. Among these genes, *Hoxa13* and *Hoxd13* in the paralog group 13 are specifically expressed in the developing distal region (the autopod). Human synpolydactyly (SPD) is a rare dominantly inherited limb malformation characterized by syndactyly between the third and fourth fingers and between the fourth and fifth toes. Typical SPD is caused by mutations of the *Hoxd13* gene such as expansions, frame-shift deletions, and functional mutations (Malik and Grzeschik, 2008). Another human malformation, the hand-foot-genital syndrome (HFGS), is associated with mutations in the *Hoxa13* gene (Goodman, 2002).

In addition, aberrant limb formation has been observed in *Hoxa13*$^{+/-}$ and *Hoxd13*$^{-/-}$ mutant mice (Dolle et al., 1993; Fromental-Ramain et al., 1996). The greater severity of the phenotypes of *Hoxa13*$^{+/-}$/*Hoxd13*$^{-/-}$ mice suggested that redundancies within paralog groups may play a role in limb development. These redundant manners are also observed in kidney formation. There are three *Hox11* paralogous genes in clusters A, C, and D. In triple mutants, metanephric induction is completely absent, and the reduction of *Six2* and *Gdnf* expression is believed to be one of the causative factors for this phenotype (Wellik et al., 2002). On the other hand, the activities of *Hox* genes within a single cluster are important for kidney formation (Di-Poi et al., 2007).

Hoxa13$^{-/-}$and *Hoxd13*$^{-/-}$ mice exhibit a reduction of branching in prostate ducts; *Hoxa13*$^{-/-}$ mutants die *in utero* with severe urinary and genital tract malformations (Podlasek et al., 1999; Podlasek et al., 1997; Warot et al., 1997). *Hoxb13* also functions in ventral prostate morphogenesis. *Hoxb13*$^{-/-}$ mice exhibit transparent ducts of the ventral prostate and these abnormalities are more severe in *Hoxb13*$^{-/-}$/*Hoxd13*$^{-/-}$ mice, which show a 50% reduction in the number of duct tips (Economides and Capecchi, 2003).

The involvement of the *Hox* genes described above in various morphogenetic events suggests the possible existence of a close relationship between *Hox* gene expression and the effects of teratogenic factors.

2.1.3 Function of *Hox* genes: Proliferation, apoptosis, and differentiation

Hox genes have different functions associated with proliferation, apoptosis, and differentiation. The *Hox* genes of the A, B, and C but not of the D clusters are transcribed in specific subpopulations during normal hematopoiesis. Gain- or loss-of-function analyses of expressed *Hox* genes showed their ability to specifically regulate different stages of hematopoietic development. Among them, *Hoxb4* serves as a positive regulator of self-renewal and expansion (engraftment) in hematopoietic stem cells (HSC) (Antonchuk et al., 2002; Kyba et al., 2002). On the other hand, definitive hematopoiesis was not disrupted in *Hoxb4*-deficient mice, but *Hoxb3*$^{-/-}$/*Hoxb4*$^{-/-}$ mice exhibited more pronounced hematopoietic differences (Bjornsson et al., 2003; Sauvageau et al., 1995). These results suggest that a more complex mechanism, such as gene redundancy, compensatory mechanisms and cross-regulatory interactions, among *Hox* genes may play a significant role in vivo.

Hox genes are involved in the regulation of cell proliferation, and their expression in tumor cells has therefore been studied. Certain *Hox* genes show aberrant expression in various tumor cells (Shah and Sukumar, 2010). These disruptions of normal *Hox* expression may affect various pathways linked to the promotion of tumorigenesis and metastasis. Moreover, some *Hox* genes (*Hoxa9, 11,* and *13*) are fusion partners of the nucleoporin gene *Nup98* in human leukemia (Moore et al., 2007). This fusion oncoprotein may play a role in modulating transcription and controls the nucleo-cytoplasmic transport of some mRNAs and proteins. Actually, the *Nup98-hox* fusion induces myeloproliferative disease and AML in mouse bone marrow transplantation models. Other fusion proteins such as *Hoxc11* or *13* are also known to induce AML.

Tumorigenesis is often characterized by alterations in the balance between proliferation and apoptosis. When viewed from this perspective, alterations in *Hox* gene expression can contribute to tumorigenesis (oncogenesis) by allowing the activation or repression of the apoptosis pathway. In breast cancer cell lines, Hoxa5 directly regulates *p53* expression by binding to its promoter (Raman et al., 2000). In addition, Hoxa5 induces apoptosis by promoting the expression of caspase 2 and caspase 8 in breast cancer cells in a p53-independent manner (Chen et al., 2004). In the fly, *Hox* genes induce the localized cell death that is essential for the maintenance of a morphological boundary between the two structures of the embryo's head, namely the maxillary and mandibular head lobes. In this case, the *Hox* gene *Deformed (Dfd)* directly activates the expression of the cell death promoting gene *reaper (rpr)*, thereby inducing localized cell death (Lohmann et al., 2002). Although it is not clear whether this apoptotic pathway is conserved in mammalian cells, some *Hox* genes show a close relationship to the apoptosis pathway.

Hox genes play crucial roles in differentiation. In HSC, the expression of *Hox* genes is downregulated during differentiation and maturation. The gain or loss of some *Hox* genes causes alterations in hematopoietic lineage commitment (He et al., 2011). Neural crest cells (NCCs) are also multipotent and can differentiate into different cell types, including peripheral and enteric neurons, glia, melanocytes, and smooth muscle. The *Hox* genes specify the location of the NCCs and contribute to the differentiation process (Minoux and Rijli, 2010).

Recent observations indicated that some *Hox* genes also have multiple functions in higher order biological mechanisms. Grooming is a stereotypic behavior in mammals and energizes the various regions of the brain, such the brainstem, striatum, and cortex. Excessive grooming manifests itself in humans as the obsessive-compulsive spectrum disorder trichtilomania. *Hoxb8* knockout mice show the excessive grooming phenotype. This abnormal behavior becomes a cause of death in knockout mice (Greer and Capecchi, 2002). Cell lineage tracing showed that this aberrant behavior can be attributed to the lack of bone marrow-derived microglia cells (Chen et al., 2010). The reduction of the total number of microglia cells in the adult brain of *Hoxb8* mutants is clear, although it remains unknown why the disruption of *Hoxb8* function only affects a small fraction of microglia cells and whether *Hoxb8* promotes the proliferation, differentiation or activation of apoptosis in a subpopulation of microglia cells.

These results indicate *Hox* genes are involved in a wide range of biological functions. However, the role of these genes in various processes is not entirely clear and knowledge of the direct targets of *Hox* genes is quite limited. We identified Hox protein target genes using chromatin immunopurification (ChIP) (Tomotsune et al., 1993). The use of modified methods, such as ChIP-sequence, is necessary to obtain further information on target genes and to understand their mechanisms of action.

2.2 *Cdx* family

The *Hox* cluster is believed to have arisen through the duplication of an ancestral ProtoHox cluster in early metazoan evolution. In this process, the ParaHox cluster genes, which show close evolutionary relationships, also arose (Garcia-Fernandez, 2005). *Cdx* (caudal-type homeo-box) genes are ParaHox genes, and three paralogous *Cdx* genes are present in the mouse genome and are located in different chromosomes. *Cdx* genes are required to correctly pattern the head to tail axis.

In *Cdx1*$^{-/-}$ mutants, an anterior homeotic transformation involving the occiput and the first three cervical vertebrae is observed. These changes are accompanied by a posterior shift of *Hox* expression involving three different clusters (Subramanian et al., 1995).

Cdx2$^{-/-}$ mutants present a much more severe phenotype and die between E3.5 and E5.5. The embryonic lethality of these mutants may be attributed to aberrations in the maturation of trophoblasts from the trophoectoderm. *Cdx2*$^{+/-}$ animals are viable but show tail abnormalities and growth retardation. Anterior homeotic transformation in the lower cervical and upper thoracic regions is also observed in skeletal analyses (Chawengsaksophak et al., 1997).

Cdx4 is an X-linked gene and no significant abnormality is observed in either sex in *Cdx4*$^{-/-}$ embryos (van Nes et al., 2006). However, double knockout *Cdx1*$^{-/-}$/*Cdx4*$^{-/0}$ mice were reported to show alterations in skeletal structure, and *Cdx2*$^{+/-}$/*Cdx4*$^{-/0}$ embryos were lethal around E10.5, which was attributed to a developmental defect of the chorio-allantoic placenta.

Cdx2$^{+/-}$/*Cdx1*$^{-/-}$ mutants show a greater degree of posterior truncation (van den Akker et al., 2002). These results indicate the existence of redundancy in the *Hox* clusters among the *Cdx* family genes. The *Cdx* family genes directly regulate some *Hox* genes, such as *Hoxa5* and *Hoxb8* (Subramanian et al., 1995; Tabaries et al., 2005), as these *Hox* genes were shown to rescue the *Cdx* mutant phenotypes (Young et al., 2009).

2.3 Another ParaHox gene

Hox and ParaHox genes belong to the ANTP class of homeobox genes. The ANTP class also includes two other genes, *Evx* (even-skipped homeotic) and *Meox* (mesenchyme homeobox). These two ParaHox genes, *Evx* and *Meox,* are located on either side of the *Hox* cluster in vertebrates. In the mouse genome, *Evx* and *Meox* each have two paralogous genes (*Evx1, Evx2, and Meox1, Meox2*) in different chromosomes. *Evx1*$^{-/-}$ is characterized by early embryonic lethality as it fails to differentiate extraembryonic tissues or to form egg cylinders (Spyropoulos and Capecchi, 1994). *Evx2*$^{-/-}$ mutants show malformation of the autopod, and these results indicate that *Evx2* has a genetic interaction with *Hoxd13* (Herault et al., 1996). *Meox1*$^{-/-}$ mutants exhibit hemi-vertebrae and rib, vertebral and cranial-vertebral fusions (Jukkola et al., 2005). *Meox2*$^{-/-}$ mutants show mild defects of rib and vertebral development (Mankoo et al., 1999).

NK (Nirenberg and Kim) homeo-box genes are evolutionary relatives of both *Hox* and ParaHox genes. In the mouse genome, there are ten *Nkx* family genes that are located in seven different chromosomes. *Nkx* family genes are mostly observed in mesodermal derivatives; in particular, *Nkx2.5* is essential for cardiac muscle differentiation (Hatcher et al., 2003).

2.4 T-box family

The T-box family genes encode a common DNA-binding domain known as the T-box and are also evolutionarily conserved transcription factors. This family of genes is composed of two independent functional domains: the T-box in the large N-terminal region and a transcriptional activation/repression domain in the C-terminal region. The *Brachyury* (or *T*) mouse mutant is characterized by a truncated tail and was discovered about 80 years ago. Until recently, 17 genes were identified as T-box family genes in vertebrates, and genetic analyses of individual genes have progressed significantly. These analyses indicate that T-box genes are widely involved in developmental processes of mesoderm specification (Naiche et al., 2005). In humans, mutations in T-box genes, including deletions, rearrangements, missense mutations, insertions, and truncation, lead to various genetic disorders (Packham and Brook, 2003). The phenotypes of T-box gene knockout mice can be compared with the phenotypes of several human genetic disorders.

Tbx1$^{-/-}$ mice have a lethal phenotype in late gestation and display a wide range of developmental abnormalities including facial abnormalities, cleft palate, cardiac outflow tract defects, and hypoplasia of the thymus and parathyroid glands (Jerome and Papaioannou, 2001; Merscher et al., 2001). In humans, chromosome 22q11 deletion syndrome is known as DiGeorge and velocardiofacial syndrome (DGS/VCFS) and its phenotypic characters include anomalies of the cardiac outflow tract, cleft palate, facial dysmophogenesis, and hypoplasia of the thymus and parathyroid glands. *Tbx1* is located in a region spanning 3 Mb, but another genes are also located in this region. *Tbx1* is thought to be a key gene in the etiology of DES/VCFS.

Tbx3$^{-/-}$ mice show a deficiency of mammary gland induction, genital abnormalities, and forelimb and hind limb malformations, and die during gestation(Davenport et al., 2003). However, *Tbx3*$^{+/-}$ mice appear fairly unaffected. Ulnar-mammary syndrome (UMS) is a pleiotropic disease associated with malformations of the posterior elements of the upper limbs, apocrine/mammary hypoplasia and/or dysfunction, dental abnormalities, and genital anomalies. Clinical manifestations are highly variable. Many similarities are exhibited in the phenotype, but gene dose sensitivities are different between humans and mice.

Tbx4$^{+/-}$mice form hind limb buds; however, they fail to outgrow them. *Tbx4*$^{-/-}$ mutants have problems with the allantoic connection to the placenta and die early in embryogenesis (Naiche and Papaioannou, 2003). The mutations in the human *Tbx4* gene are linked to an autosomal dominant disorder called small patella syndrome (SPS) (Bongers et al., 2004).

Tbx5$^{-/-}$ resulted in early embryonic lethality due to severe defects in early heart formation (Bruneau et al., 2001). Holt-Oram syndrome is an autosomal dominant disorder that includes cardiac and upper limb malformations. *Tbx5*$^{+/-}$ mutants faithfully recapitulate the human phenotype, including cardiac defects and forelimb malformations.

As *Tbx19* (known as *Tpit*) expression is restricted to the pituitary gland, *Tbx19*$^{-/-}$ mutants show a significant reduction in the number of pituitary POMC (pro-opiomelanocortin)-expressing cells (Pulichino et al., 2003). In humans, the absence of pituitary POMC leads to a lack of adrenocorticotrophin (ACTH), resulting in adrenal insufficiency.

The *Tbx22*$^{-/-}$ mutation caused death within 24 hr after birth due to submucous cleft palate and ankyloglossia (Pauws et al., 2009). In humans, *Tbx22* is a gene responsible for X-linked cleft palate and ankyloglossia (Braybrook et al., 2001).

3. Developmental toxicants

Teratology is the study of abnormal development and congenital malformations attributed to genetic factors, maternal factors, toxicants, or other factors such as environmental chemicals. In the early 1970s, James G. Wilson created "The Six Principles of Teratology". These principles are still applied today and guide the investigation of teratogenic agents and their effects on the development of organisms. A wide variety of chemicals and environmental factors are believed to have teratogenic potential in humans and animals. In the USA, the Food and Drug Administration (FDA) has categorized drugs into five different risk categories for pregnant women. These five categories (A, B, C, D, and X) have been considered a therapeutic advantage but they are only based on specific criteria and are not universal. Therefore, the number of these factors is likely higher than one thousand and is increasing daily. The teratogenic potentials of various chemicals and environmental factors are determined using animal models (e.g., zebra fish, mouse, rat, pig, rabbit, dog, and monkey). In the past, observations of the characteristics of embryos from candidate-exposed pregnant animals were used as the main criteria, but current teratological evaluations need to include knowledge about the molecular mechanisms.

In this section, six xenobiotics known to be developmental toxicants in humans were selected for further description.

3.1 Endocrine disruptors

Under normal conditions, hormones are involved in the maintenance of homeostasis, but endocrine disruptors, which are environmental chemicals that have a hormone action or inhibit the activity of an endogenous hormone, have an adverse effect on organs and progeny. In adults, the role of the endocrine system in the maintenance of homeostasis is established and adults therefore have resistance against endocrine disruptors. However, in the fetus, infants, and children, resistance against these agents may be weak and they therefore can have irreversible impact on developmental functions such as organ formation.

Endocrine disruptors are found in low doses in products of daily use. DTT, polychlorinated biphenyls (PCBs), bisphenol A (BPA), polybrominated diphenyl esters (PBDEs), and a variety of phthalates are chemicals used in pesticides, plastic food containers or plastic toys, and are currently recognized as endocrine disruptors.

Methoxychlor (MXC) is an organochlorine DDT derivative. MXC was shown to affect fertility in mice and cause maternal weight gain in fetal rats. These effects are thought to be mediated by the inhibition of estrogen binding to the Estrogen Receptor (Esr), by MXC and the suppression of the expression of *Hoxa10* (Fei et al., 2005).

BPA also affects estrogen signaling. In BPA-exposed males, an increase in the size of the prostate gland and oligospermia are observed. BPA exposure negatively regulates the expression of *Hoxa10* and *Hoxa11* and affects estrogen signaling (Varayoud et al., 2008).

Estrogen and androgen are sex steroids that are needed for the proper development of reproductive organs (Dupont et al., 2000). Each steroid binds to a specific nuclear-receptor and these receptors act as ligand-dependent transcription factors. Alterations in *Hox* gene expression induced by endocrine disruptors is thus considered to be a nuclear receptor-mediated mechanism.

3.2 Diethylstilbestrol (DES)

DES is a synthetic nonsteroidal estrogen. This chemical was used as a pharmaceutical product for the prevention of miscarriage in the 1970s, but vaginal cancer occurred frequently in children whose mothers took DES. Exposed offspring also experienced a high incidence of pregnancy wastage and preterm labor. DES induced altered *Hox* gene expression in human uterine endometrial and cervical cells. In reproductive organs, *Hox* genes are also expressed along the A-P axis. Under this rule, *Hoxa9* is normally expressed in the oviduct and *Hoxa10* in the uterus. However, this linear regulation of expression is disrupted in DES-exposed humans or mice, and the expressional domain is shifted posteriorly (Block et al., 2000). DES binds the Esr, and the irregular nuclear receptor activation may lead to aberrant *Hox* gene expression.

3.3 Anticonvulsants (VPA)

Valoproic acid (VPA) is a chemical compound used for the treatment of epilepsy. However, VPA has teratogenic potential along with other anticonvulsant drugs, including carbamazepine and phenytoin in humans. Having weak developmental toxicant of carbamazepine and phenytoin, VPA exposure is more toxicant. In humans, infants exposed to VPA *in utero* show anomalies including neural, craniofacial, cardiovascular, and skeletal defects. A similar teratology is exhibited in rodents, rabbits, and nonhuman primates. The spina bifida, a neural tube defect, is also observed in VPA-exposed infants at frequencies of 1–2%. VPA exposed human embryonic carcinoma (NTera2/D1) cells show slight alterations in the expression of certain *Hox* genes (Faiella et al., 2000). VPA is also an inhibitor of class I and IIa HDACs (histone deacetylases); therefore, changes in the expressions of various genes are thought to occur in different tissues. However, it remains largely unknown why phenotypes appear only in limited organs in which HDAC is the primary target of VPA, and the mechanisms underlying the action of VPA are not clear.

3.4 Thalidomide

Thalidomide (α-phthaliidoglutarimide) was used as a sedative and for morning sickness in the late 1950s. However, reports of the teratogenic potency of thalidomide appeared in the early 1960s. In these reports, infants exposed to thalidomide during the early stages of pregnancy had multiple defects, such as malformations of the limbs, ears, eyes, internal organs and central nervous system. The most commonly observed defects were limb malformations including amelia (complete absence of the limb) and phocomelia (truncation or absence of the zeugopod). Thalidomide-induced limb defects are observed in humans, monkeys, rabbits and chicks, but these phenotypes are not observed in the mouse or rat (Vargesson, 2009). For 50 years, the mechanism of thalidomide-teratogenicity was poorly understood. Thalidomide is a derivative of glutamic acid and contains two imide rings: glutarimide and phthalimide. Thalidomide has therefore been believed to act by causing biochemical alterations of glutamic acid, nucleic acids and vitamin B. Recently, the primary target of thalidomide was identified and parts of the molecular mechanism were revealed (Ito et al., 2010). A thalidomide-binding protein, *Cereblon* (CRBN), forms an E3 ubiquitin ligase complex with Ddb1 and Cul4A in a thalidomide-dependent manner and modifies the expression of *Fgf8* in the limb. Generally, the limb has three developmental axes: the proximal-distal axis, which runs from the base of the limb to the tip; the A-P axis, which runs parallel with the body axis; and the D-V axis, which runs from the back of the hand to the palm. Under the control of these three axes, various positional identities are specified by the concentration gradient of diffusible factors, such as *Fgfs*, *Bmps*, *Wnt*, and *Sonic Hedgehog*. The malformed fin or limb in knockdown *Crbn* zebrafish or the dominant negative form of *Crbn* expressing chicken, respectively, indicated the important role of the ubiquitin ligase pathway for morphogenesis through thalidomide, and clearly showed that the reduction of *Fgf8* expression lead to the deformity of the limb. Although there is no information about the specific target molecule of *Crbn,* identification of this target molecule will allow a more effective use of thalidomide for the treatment of multiple myeloma and erythema nodosum leprosum and avoid its associated teratogenic risks.

3.5 Retinoic acid

In normal embryogenesis, a wide variety of diffusible factors act as morphogens and control proper morphogenesis. Retinoic acid is one of the morphogens that function during the formation of various organs such as the head, trunk, limbs, heart, and the central nervous system. Retinol and other retinoid compounds, which are precursors of retinoic acid, cannot be synthesized *de novo* and must therefore be ingested in food or supplements. After modification of ingested retinol by multiple enzymes, the resulting compounds bind to ligand-activated nuclear receptors, namely Rar (retinoic acid receptor) and Rxr (retinoid X receptor). *Rar* and *Rxr* are concurrently encoded by three family genes (α, β, and γ), and subtypes exist that are products of alternative splicing or different promoter usage. The activated nuclear receptors form homo- or hetero-dimers and recruit coactivators or corepressors to the RARE (retinoic acid response element) on the target genes. Some target genes have been identified and these genes function in the cell cycle, proliferation, and morphogenesis (Delacroix et al., 2010; Nielsen et al., 2008).

Retinoids were found to be teratogenic in humans in the early 1980s. Infants exposed during gestation have teratogenic syndrome including craniofacial abnormalities and defects of the thymic, cardiovascular, and central nervous system. The teratogenic effect is observed in other animal models, such as mouse, rat, pig, rabbit, dog, chick, and monkey. The dosage and timing of gestational exposure profoundly influence the form of the birth defect and the lethality, but differences in the genetic background in mice also have an effect. The peak period of sensitivity for a given tissue appears to be during the development of the primordial structures.

Rar and *Rxr* knockout mice were produced by several methods and these mice exhibited various phenotypes (Mark et al., 2006). However, their abnormalities were restricted to a subset of tissues normally expressing these receptors, probably reflecting the existence of functional redundancies between nuclear receptors. The expression of certain *Hox* genes is controlled via RARE (Oosterveen et al., 2003). Although differences in the RA exposure dosage determine the phenotypes, aberrant *Hox* gene expression is thought to play a role in the morphological malformations.

3.6 Dioxin

PCDDs (polychlorinated dibenzo-p-dioxins), PCDFs (polychlorinated dibenzofurans) and DL-PCBs (dioxin-like polychlorinated biphenyls) are generically termed as dioxin and are similar toxicants. Dioxin is an environmental contaminant and is unintentionally generated as a by-product of industrial combustion. Among dioxins, TCDD (2, 3, 7, 8-Tetrachlorodibenzo-p-dioxin) is the most severe toxicant and has the highest teratogenic potency in mammals. Differences in the exposure dosage determine the resulting phenotypes, which include cleft palate, hydronephrosis, and defects of sex organs. There are differences due to timing and dose of exposure, TCDD exposure causes a significant decrease in ventral prostate development, which is similar to the effect of impairment of certain *Hox* genes (Vezina et al., 2009), but the correlativity between TCDD and *Hox* expression is not cleared.

The molecular mechanisms of the xenobiotic dioxin pathway can be understood through the analyses of nuclear receptors. The toxicant and teratogenic effects of dioxin are thought to depend on the activation of the Ahr (aryl hydorocarbon receptor) pathway. Ahr has multiple functions. Ahr is a ligand-activated transcription factor that is a member of the bHLH/PAS (basic Helix-loop-Helix/Per-Arnt-Sim) family of genes. Ahr generally localizes to the cytoplasm and forms a complex with Hsp90 (heat shock protein 90), cochaperone p23, and the immunophilin-like protein Ara9 (Bell and Poland, 2000). Upon binding ligand, Ahr is released from the p23/Ara9 complex and translocates to the nucleus. In the nucleus, Ahr dissociates from Hsp90 and dimerizes with another bHLH-PAS family gene, Arnt (Ahr nuclear translocator). The Ahr/Arnt heterodimer binds to specific DNA sequences termed XREs (xenobiotic response elements: 5′-GCGTG-3′) and regulates target gene expression with transcriptional coactivators/corepressors, which are also partners of Rar/Rxr (Beischlag et al., 2002). Currently, various genes are reported as Ahr target genes: phase I drug metabolizing enzymes, such as those of the *Cyp450* (Cytochorome 450) family; phase II enzymes, such as *Ugt1a1* (Kohle and Bock, 2007); and as down stream genes of Ahr-pathway, such as cytokines, and *Tgf* family which are unrelated xenobiotic metabolism genes (Haarmann-Stemmann et al., 2009).

Ahr is also a modulator of estrogen receptor signaling. Ohtake et al. indicated that the ligand-activated Ahr/Arnt heterodimer directly associates with the Esr, recruits a coactivator, and regulates the expression of Esr target genes (Ohtake et al., 2003). In this case, Ahr functions as activator/repressor depending on the ligand binding state of the Esr. Another function of ligand-activated Ahr as a substrate-specific adaptor in the Cullin 4B ubiquitin ligase complex was described (Ohtake et al., 2007). In this case, agonist (3MC: 3-methylcholanthrene)-activated Ahr ubiquitinates Esr1 and androgen receptor (Ar) in vitro and in vivo. In *Ahr*-deficient mice, responses to dioxin such as the induction of *Cyp1a1* activation were not observed. However, null mutants have functional impairments of male and female reproductive organs, depending on the affected allele (Schmidt et al., 1996). Although there are other identified ligands for Ahr, including flavonoids, UV photo-products of tryptophan and some synthetic retinoids, the above observations suggest that Ahr plays a role in the cross talk between the dioxin and RA pathways.

4. Hox-RA/dioxin

The identification of molecular markers for the variety of existing teratogenic factors is an urgent need in various respects. In the present report, we focused on the expressional changes of the *Hox* cluster genes in embryos exposed to teratogenic factors because their aberrant expression lead to various morphological defects and the affected animals have close similarities (Kojima and Takahashi, 2009).

Because the different amount and timing of exposure to teratogenic factors are correlated to the different effects in embryos, we firstly examined the RA or dioxin effects in E10.5 embryos for 6 hr by one-shot administration. This dose induced craniofacial and skeletal defects in RA-exposed embryos, and hydronephrosis in dioxin-exposed embryos. Among 39 *Hox* cluster genes, 3′-located paralogs (*Hox1~8*) were up-regulated and some 5′-located genes (*Hoxa11, Hoxd9, and Hoxd12*) were down-regulated in the RA-exposed embryos (*Fig. 1*). Meanwhile, the influence of relative position in the cluster was not observed in the TCDD-exposed embryos. A and D cluster genes were down-regulated and no clear difference was observed in the cluster B. Additionally, aberrant expression of pri-miRNAs (precursors of miRNAs) was detected (*Fig. 2*). These pri-miRNA changes were correlated with changes in the expression of closely located *Hox* genes.

TCDD exposure causes a decrease in the levels of all-trans RA in the liver, which is the main RA storage location in a variety of species (Fletcher et al., 2001). There are some similarities in terms of morphological changes between RA- and TCDD-exposed embryos. The developmental effects of the replacement of RA storage by TCDD are not clear, but it is suggested that TCDD and related compounds have an impact on retinoid homeostasis and the RA signaling pathway. Our analyses indicate that alterations in the expression of *Hox* cluster genes do not show a clear correlation with these teratogenic factors. In addition, expressional changes of some pri-miRNAs in the *Hox* clusters are also different between these two factors. Although the involvement of Ahr in the cross talk between the RA and TCDD pathways is possible, there are clear differences in the downstream effects, such as expressional changes of *Hox* cluster genes. We also detected changes in the expression of other transcription factors, such as ParaHoxs and T-box family genes, in embryos exposed to these factors. Some genes show a specific response to each teratogenic factor. Based on these results, changes in the expression of transcription factors can be considered as potential molecular markers for the verification of teratogenic effects. Therefore, to better determine the teratogenic potential of various chemicals, further investigation of the effects of the timing or dosage of RA and TCDD in exposed embryos is under way.

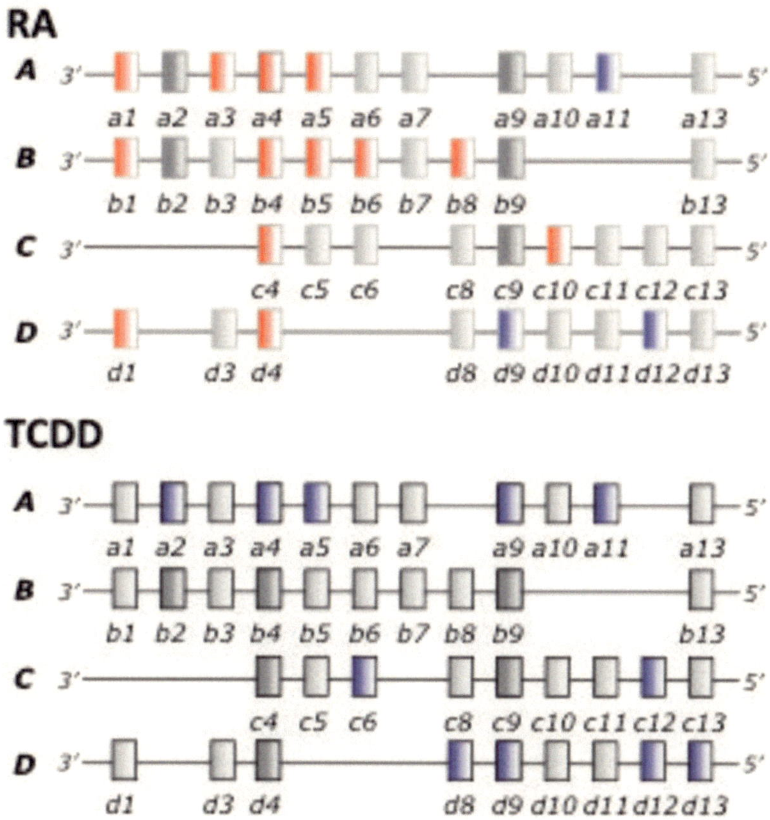

Fig. 1. Expressional changes of the *Hox* cluster genes in embryos treated with teratogenic agents. 39 *Hox* genes are separated on four clusters (A, B, C, and D) in four chromosomal loci. The box indicates each gene. Red boxes indicate up-regulated and blue boxes indicate down-regulated genes in response to treatment with teratogenic agents.

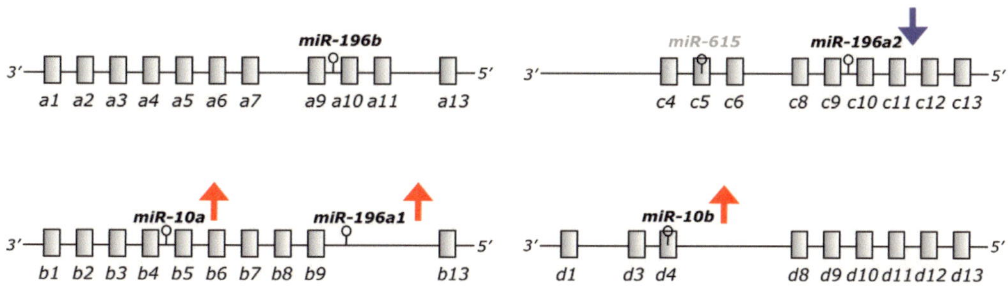

Fig. 2. Expressional changes of pri-miRNAs in the *Hox* cluster genes. Three miRNA family genes (*miR-196, miR-10, and miR-615*) are located in the *Hox* cluster. Red arrows indicate RA and the blue arrow indicates TCDD exposure. The upward direction of the arrow represents increased expression and the downward direction represents decreased expression.

5. Conclusions

Contrasting a comprehensive analysis using DNA microarrays, our analysis is simpler and allows the examination of a large number of samples. Information on molecular markers such as the *Hox* genes under various conditions (exposure-time, -dosage) will allow the prediction of the hazardous nature of unknown factors. In addition, the understanding of the molecular mechanisms common to different teratogenic agents requires the identification of the target genes of Hox protein and each transcription factor and an understanding of transcription factor networks.

6. References

Antonchuk, J., Sauvageau, G., and Humphries, R.K. (2002). HOXB4-induced expansion of adult hematopoietic stem cells ex vivo. *Cell* 109, 39-45.

Augui, S., Nora, E.P., and Heard, E. (2011). Regulation of X-chromosome inactivation by the X-inactivation centre. *Nat Rev Genet* 12, 429-442.

Balling, R., Mutter, G., Gruss, P., and Kessel, M. (1989). Craniofacial abnormalities induced by ectopic expression of the homeobox gene Hox-1.1 in transgenic mice. *Cell* 58, 337-347.

Beischlag, T.V., Wang, S., Rose, D.W., Torchia, J., Reisz-Porszasz, S., Muhammad, K., Nelson, W.E., Probst, M.R., Rosenfeld, M.G., and Hankinson, O. (2002). Recruitment of the NCoA/SRC-1/p160 family of transcriptional coactivators by the aryl hydrocarbon receptor/aryl hydrocarbon receptor nuclear translocator complex. *Mol.Cell.Biol.* 22, 4319-4333.

Bell, D.R., and Poland, A. (2000). Binding of aryl hydrocarbon receptor (AhR) to AhR-interacting protein. The role of hsp90. *J Biol Chem* 275, 36407-36414.

Bernstein, B.E., Mikkelsen, T.S., Xie, X., Kamal, M., Huebert, D.J., Cuff, J., Fry, B., Meissner, A., Wernig, M., Plath, K., *et al.* (2006). A bivalent chromatin structure marks key developmental genes in embryonic stem cells. *Cell* 125, 315-326.

Bjornsson, J.M., Larsson, N., Brun, A.C., Magnusson, M., Andersson, E., Lundstrom, P., Larsson, J., Repetowska, E., Ehinger, M., Humphries, R.K., *et al.* (2003). Reduced proliferative capacity of hematopoietic stem cells deficient in Hoxb3 and Hoxb4. *Mol.Cell.Biol.* 23, 3872-3883.

Block, K., Kardana, A., Igarashi, P., and Taylor, H.S. (2000). In utero diethylstilbestrol (DES) exposure alters Hox gene expression in the developing mullerian system. *Faseb J* 14, 1101-1108.

Bongers, E.M., Duijf, P.H., van Beersum, S.E., Schoots, J., Van Kampen, A., Burckhardt, A., Hamel, B.C., Losan, F., Hoefsloot, L.H., Yntema, H.G., *et al.* (2004). Mutations in the human TBX4 gene cause small patella syndrome. *Am. J. Hum. Genet.* 74, 1239-1248.

Braybrook, C., Doudney, K., Marcano, A.C., Arnason, A., Bjornsson, A., Patton, M.A., Goodfellow, P.J., Moore, G.E., and Stanier, P. (2001). The T-box transcription factor gene TBX22 is mutated in X-linked cleft palate and ankyloglossia. *Nat Genet* 29, 179-183.

Bruneau, B.G., Nemer, G., Schmitt, J.P., Charron, F., Robitaille, L., Caron, S., Conner, D.A., Gessler, M., Nemer, M., Seidman, C.E., *et al.* (2001). A murine model of Holt-Oram syndrome defines roles of the T-box transcription factor Tbx5 in cardiogenesis and disease. *Cell* 106, 709-721.

Chawengsaksophak, K., James, R., Hammond, V.E., Kontgen, F., and Beck, F. (1997). Homeosis and intestinal tumours in Cdx2 mutant mice. *Nature* 386, 84-87.

Chen, H., Chung, S., and Sukumar, S. (2004). HOXA5-induced apoptosis in breast cancer cells is mediated by caspases 2 and 8. *Mol. Cell. Biol.* 24, 924-935.

Chen, S.K., Tvrdik, P., Peden, E., Cho, S., Wu, S., Spangrude, G., and Capecchi, M.R. (2010). Hematopoietic origin of pathological grooming in Hoxb8 mutant mice. *Cell* 141, 775-785.

Davenport, T.G., Jerome-Majewska, L.A., and Papaioannou, V.E. (2003). Mammary gland, limb and yolk sac defects in mice lacking Tbx3, the gene mutated in human ulnar mammary syndrome. *Development* 130, 2263-2273.

Delacroix, L., Moutier, E., Altobelli, G., Legras, S., Poch, O., Choukrallah, M.A., Bertin, I., Jost, B., and Davidson, I. (2010). Cell-specific interaction of retinoic acid receptors with target genes in mouse embryonic fibroblasts and embryonic stem cells. *Mol.Cell.Biol.* 30, 231-244.

Di-Poi, N., Zakany, J., and Duboule, D. (2007). Distinct roles and regulations for HoxD genes in metanephric kidney development. *PLoS Genet* 3, e232.

Dolle, P., Dierich, A., LeMeur, M., Schimmang, T., Schuhbaur, B., Chambon, P., and Duboule, D. (1993). Disruption of the Hoxd-13 gene induces localized heterochrony leading to mice with neotenic limbs. *Cell* 75, 431-441.

Dupont, S., Krust, A., Gansmuller, A., Dierich, A., Chambon, P., and Mark, M. (2000). Effect of single and compound knockouts of estrogen receptors alpha (ERalpha) and beta (ERbeta) on mouse reproductive phenotypes. *Development* 127, 4277-4291.

Economides, K.D., and Capecchi, M.R. (2003). Hoxb13 is required for normal differentiation and secretory function of the ventral prostate. *Development* 130, 2061-2069.

Faiella, A., Wernig, M., Consalez, G.G., Hostick, U., Hofmann, C., Hustert, E., Boncinelli, E., Balling, R., and Nadeau, J.H. (2000). A mouse model for valproate teratogenicity: parental effects, homeotic transformations, and altered HOX expression. *Hum. Mol. Genet.* 9, 227-236.

Fei, X., Chung, H., and Taylor, H.S. (2005). Methoxychlor disrupts uterine Hoxa10 gene expression. *Endocrinology* 146, 3445-3451.

Fletcher, N., Hanberg, A., and Hakansson, H. (2001). Hepatic vitamin a depletion is a sensitive marker of 2,3,7,8-tetrachlorodibenzo-p-dioxin (TCDD) exposure in four rodent species. *Toxicol Sci* 62, 166-175.

Fromental-Ramain, C., Warot, X., Messadecq, N., LeMeur, M., Dolle, P., and Chambon, P. (1996). Hoxa-13 and Hoxd-13 play a crucial role in the patterning of the limb autopod. *Development* 122, 2997-3011.

Garcia-Fernandez, J. (2005). The genesis and evolution of homeobox gene clusters. *Nat Rev Genet* 6, 881-892.

Gendron-Maguire, M., Mallo, M., Zhang, M., and Gridley, T. (1993). Hoxa-2 mutant mice exhibit homeotic transformation of skeletal elements derived from cranial neural crest. *Cell* 75, 1317-1331.

Goodman, F.R. (2002). Limb malformations and the human HOX genes. *Am. J. Med. Genet.* 112, 256-265.

Greer, J.M., and Capecchi, M.R. (2002). Hoxb8 is required for normal grooming behavior in mice. *Neuron* 33, 23-34.

Haarmann-Stemmann, T., Bothe, H., and Abel, J. (2009). Growth factors, cytokines and their receptors as downstream targets of arylhydrocarbon receptor (AhR) signaling pathways. *Biochem Pharmacol* 77, 508-520.

Hatcher, C.J., Diman, N.Y., McDermott, D.A., and Basson, C.T. (2003). Transcription factor cascades in congenital heart malformation. *Trends. Mol. Med.* 9, 512-515.

He, H., Hua, X., and Yan, J. (2011). Epigenetic regulations in hematopoietic Hox code. *Oncogene* 30, 379-388.

Herault, Y., Hraba-Renevey, S., van der Hoeven, F., and Duboule, D. (1996). Function of the Evx-2 gene in the morphogenesis of vertebrate limbs. *EMBO J* 15, 6727-6738.

Hornstein, E., Mansfield, J.H., Yekta, S., Hu, J.K., Harfe, B.D., McManus, M.T., Baskerville, S., Bartel, D.P., and Tabin, C.J. (2005). The microRNA miR-196 acts upstream of Hoxb8 and Shh in limb development. *Nature* 438, 671-674.

Hughes, C.L., and Kaufman, T.C. (2002). Hox genes and the evolution of the arthropod body plan. *Evol Dev* 4, 459-499.

Ito, T., Ando, H., Suzuki, T., Ogura, T., Hotta, K., Imamura, Y., Yamaguchi, Y., and Handa, H. (2010). Identification of a primary target of thalidomide teratogenicity. *Science* 327, 1345-1350.

Jerome, L.A., and Papaioannou, V.E. (2001). DiGeorge syndrome phenotype in mice mutant for the T-box gene, Tbx1. *Nat Genet* 27, 286-291.

Jukkola, T., Trokovic, R., Maj, P., Lamberg, A., Mankoo, B., Pachnis, V., Savilahti, H., and Partanen, J. (2005). Meox1Cre: a mouse line expressing Cre recombinase in somitic mesoderm. *Genesis* 43, 148-153.

Kohle, C., and Bock, K.W. (2007). Coordinate regulation of Phase I and II xenobiotic metabolisms by the Ah receptor and Nrf2. *Biochem Pharmacol* 73, 1853-1862.

Kojima, T., and Takahashi, N. (2009). Influence of teratogenic factors on mouse 39 hox gene expression. *Biosci. Biotechnol. Biochem.* 73, 2416-2421.

Kyba, M., Perlingeiro, R.C., and Daley, G.Q. (2002). HoxB4 confers definitive lymphoid-myeloid engraftment potential on embryonic stem cell and yolk sac hematopoietic progenitors. *Cell* 109, 29-37.

Lohmann, I., McGinnis, N., Bodmer, M., and McGinnis, W. (2002). The Drosophila Hox gene deformed sculpts head morphology via direct regulation of the apoptosis activator reaper. *Cell* 110, 457-466.

Malik, S., and Grzeschik, K.H. (2008). Synpolydactyly: clinical and molecular advances. *Clin Genet* 73, 113-120.

Mallo, M., Wellik, D.M., and Deschamps, J. (2010). Hox genes and regional patterning of the vertebrate body plan. *Dev Biol* 344, 7-15.

Mankoo, B.S., Collins, N.S., Ashby, P., Grigorieva, E., Pevny, L.H., Candia, A., Wright, C.V., Rigby, P.W., and Pachnis, V. (1999). Mox2 is a component of the genetic hierarchy controlling limb muscle development. *Nature* 400, 69-73.

Mansfield, J.H., Harfe, B.D., Nissen, R., Obenauer, J., Srineel, J., Chaudhuri, A., Farzan-Kashani, R., Zuker, M., Pasquinelli, A.E., Ruvkun, G., *et al.* (2004). MicroRNA-responsive 'sensor' transgenes uncover Hox-like and other developmentally regulated patterns of vertebrate microRNA expression. *Nat Genet* 36, 1079-1083.

Mark, M., Ghyselinck, N.B., and Chambon, P. (2006). Function of retinoid nuclear receptors: lessons from genetic and pharmacological dissections of the retinoic acid signaling pathway during mouse embryogenesis. *Annu. Rev. Pharmacol. Toxicol.* 46, 451-480.

McLain, K., Schreiner, C., Yager, K.L., Stock, J.L., and Potter, S.S. (1992). Ectopic expression of Hox-2.3 induces craniofacial and skeletal malformations in transgenic mice. *Mech Dev* 39, 3-16.

Mendenhall, E.M., and Bernstein, B.E. (2008). Chromatin state maps: new technologies, new insights. *Curr. Opin. Genet. Dev.* 18, 109-115.

Merscher, S., Funke, B., Epstein, J.A., Heyer, J., Puech, A., Lu, M.M., Xavier, R.J., Demay, M.B., Russell, R.G., Factor, S., *et al.* (2001). TBX1 is responsible for cardiovascular defects in velo-cardio-facial/DiGeorge syndrome. *Cell* 104, 619-629.

Minoux, M., and Rijli, F.M. (2010). Molecular mechanisms of cranial neural crest cell migration and patterning in craniofacial development. *Development* 137, 2605-2621.

Moens, C.B., and Selleri, L. (2006). Hox cofactors in vertebrate development. *Dev Biol* 291, 193-206.

Moore, M.A., Chung, K.Y., Plasilova, M., Schuringa, J.J., Shieh, J.H., Zhou, P., and Morrone, G. (2007). NUP98 dysregulation in myeloid leukemogenesis. *Ann. N. Y. Acad. Sci.* 1106, 114-142.

Naiche, L.A., Harrelson, Z., Kelly, R.G., and Papaioannou, V.E. (2005). T-box genes in vertebrate development. *Annu Rev Genet* 39, 219-239.

Naiche, L.A., and Papaioannou, V.E. (2003). Loss of Tbx4 blocks hindlimb development and affects vascularization and fusion of the allantois. *Development* 130, 2681-2693.

Nielsen, R., Pedersen, T.A., Hagenbeek, D., Moulos, P., Siersbaek, R., Megens, E., Denissov, S., Borgesen, M., Francoijs, K.J., Mandrup, S., *et al.* (2008). Genome-wide profiling of PPARgamma:RXR and RNA polymerase II occupancy reveals temporal activation of distinct metabolic pathways and changes in RXR dimer composition during adipogenesis. *Genes Dev* 22, 2953-2967.

Ohtake, F., Baba, A., Takada, I., Okada, M., Iwasaki, K., Miki, H., Takahashi, S., Kouzmenko, A., Nohara, K., Chiba, T., *et al.* (2007). Dioxin receptor is a ligand-dependent E3 ubiquitin ligase. *Nature* 446, 562-566.

Ohtake, F., Takeyama, K., Matsumoto, T., Kitagawa, H., Yamamoto, Y., Nohara, K., Tohyama, C., Krust, A., Mimura, J., Chambon, P., *et al.* (2003). Modulation of oestrogen receptor signalling by association with the activated dioxin receptor. *Nature* 423, 545-550.

Oosterveen, T., Niederreither, K., Dolle, P., Chambon, P., Meijlink, F., and Deschamps, J. (2003). Retinoids regulate the anterior expression boundaries of 5' Hoxb genes in posterior hindbrain. *EMBO J* 22, 262-269.

Packham, E.A., and Brook, J.D. (2003). T-box genes in human disorders. *Hum. Mol. Genet.* 12 Spec No 1, R37-44.

Pauws, E., Hoshino, A., Bentley, L., Prajapati, S., Keller, C., Hammond, P., Martinez-Barbera, J.P., Moore, G.E., and Stanier, P. (2009). Tbx22null mice have a submucous cleft palate due to reduced palatal bone formation and also display ankyloglossia and choanal atresia phenotypes. *Hum. Mol. Genet.* 18, 4171-4179.

Podlasek, C.A., Clemens, J.Q., and Bushman, W. (1999). Hoxa-13 gene mutation results in abnormal seminal vesicle and prostate development. *J Urol* 161, 1655-1661.

Podlasek, C.A., Duboule, D., and Bushman, W. (1997). Male accessory sex organ morphogenesis is altered by loss of function of Hoxd-13. *Dev Dyn* 208, 454-465.

Pulichino, A.M., Vallette-Kasic, S., Tsai, J.P., Couture, C., Gauthier, Y., and Drouin, J. (2003). Tpit determines alternate fates during pituitary cell differentiation. *Genes Dev* 17, 738-747.

Raman, V., Martensen, S.A., Reisman, D., Evron, E., Odenwald, W.F., Jaffee, E., Marks, J., and Sukumar, S. (2000). Compromised HOXA5 function can limit p53 expression in human breast tumours. *Nature* 405, 974-978.

Rinn, J.L., Kertesz, M., Wang, J.K., Squazzo, S.L., Xu, X., Brugmann, S.A., Goodnough, L.H., Helms, J.A., Farnham, P.J., Segal, E., *et al.* (2007). Functional demarcation of active and silent chromatin domains in human HOX loci by noncoding RNAs. *Cell* 129, 1311-1323.

Sauvageau, G., Thorsteinsdottir, U., Eaves, C.J., Lawrence, H.J., Largman, C., Lansdorp, P.M., and Humphries, R.K. (1995). Overexpression of HOXB4 in hematopoietic cells causes the selective expansion of more primitive populations in vitro and in vivo. *Genes Dev* 9, 1753-1765.

Schmidt, J.V., Su, G.H., Reddy, J.K., Simon, M.C., and Bradfield, C.A. (1996). Characterization of a murine Ahr null allele: involvement of the Ah receptor in hepatic growth and development. *Proc. Natl. Acad. Sci. USA* 93, 6731-6736.

Shah, N., and Sukumar, S. (2010). The Hox genes and their roles in oncogenesis. *Nat Rev Cancer* 10, 361-371.

Spyropoulos, D.D., and Capecchi, M.R. (1994). Targeted disruption of the even-skipped gene, evx1, causes early postimplantation lethality of the mouse conceptus. *Genes Dev* 8, 1949-1961.

Subramanian, V., Meyer, B.I., and Gruss, P. (1995). Disruption of the murine homeobox gene Cdx1 affects axial skeletal identities by altering the mesodermal expression domains of Hox genes. *Cell* 83, 641-653.

Tabaries, S., Lapointe, J., Besch, T., Carter, M., Woollard, J., Tuggle, C.K., and Jeannotte, L. (2005). Cdx protein interaction with Hoxa5 regulatory sequences contributes to Hoxa5 regional expression along the axial skeleton. *Mol.Cell.Biol.* 25, 1389-1401.

Tomotsune, D., Shoji, H., Wakamatsu, Y., Kondoh, H., and Takahashi, N. (1993). A mouse homologue of the Drosophila tumour-suppressor gene l(2)gl controlled by Hox-C8 in vivo. *Nature* 365, 69-72.

van den Akker, E., Forlani, S., Chawengsaksophak, K., de Graaff, W., Beck, F., Meyer, B.I., and Deschamps, J. (2002). Cdx1 and Cdx2 have overlapping functions in anteroposterior patterning and posterior axis elongation. *Development* 129, 2181-2193.

van Nes, J., de Graaff, W., Lebrin, F., Gerhard, M., Beck, F., and Deschamps, J. (2006). The Cdx4 mutation affects axial development and reveals an essential role of Cdx genes in the ontogenesis of the placental labyrinth in mice. *Development* 133, 419-428.

Varayoud, J., Ramos, J.G., Bosquiazzo, V.L., Munoz-de-Toro, M., and Luque, E.H. (2008). Developmental exposure to Bisphenol a impairs the uterine response to ovarian steroids in the adult. *Endocrinology* 149, 5848-5860.

Vargesson, N. (2009). Thalidomide-induced limb defects: resolving a 50-year-old puzzle. *Bioessays* 31, 1327-1336.

Vezina, C.M., Lin, T.M., and Peterson, R.E. (2009). AHR signaling in prostate growth, morphogenesis, and disease. *Biochem Pharmacol* 77, 566-576.

Wang, K.C., Yang, Y.W., Liu, B., Sanyal, A., Corces-Zimmerman, R., Chen, Y., Lajoie, B.R., Protacio, A., Flynn, R.A., Gupta, R.A., *et al.* (2011). A long noncoding RNA maintains active chromatin to coordinate homeotic gene expression. *Nature* 472, 120-124.

Warot, X., Fromental-Ramain, C., Fraulob, V., Chambon, P., and Dolle, P. (1997). Gene dosage-dependent effects of the Hoxa-13 and Hoxd-13 mutations on morphogenesis of the terminal parts of the digestive and urogenital tracts. *Development* 124, 4781-4791.

Wellik, D.M. (2009). Hox genes and vertebrate axial pattern. *Curr. Top. Dev. Biol.* 88, 257-278.

Wellik, D.M., Hawkes, P.J., and Capecchi, M.R. (2002). Hox11 paralogous genes are essential for metanephric kidney induction. *Genes Dev* 16, 1423-1432.

Yekta, S., Shih, I.H., and Bartel, D.P. (2004). MicroRNA-directed cleavage of HOXB8 mRNA. *Science* 304, 594-596.

Young, T., Rowland, J.E., van de Ven, C., Bialecka, M., Novoa, A., Carapuco, M., van Nes, J., de Graaff, W., Duluc, I., Freund, J.N., *et al.* (2009). Cdx and Hox genes differentially regulate posterior axial growth in mammalian embryos. *Dev Cell* 17, 516-526.

2

Signalling Mechanisms Underlying Congenital Malformation: The Gatekeepers, Glypicans

Annalisa Fico[1,2] and Rosanna Dono[1]
[1]*Developmental Biology Institute of Marseille-Luminy CNRS UMR 6216,*
[2]*Institute of Genetics and Biophisics, CNR,*
[1]*France*
[2]*Italy*

1. Introduction

Congenital malformations contribute to a significant proportion of infant morbidity and remain a leading cause of death in both the neonatal and postneonatal periods (Brunner and van Driel, 2004). Despite the high frequency of these disorders, their underlying causes remain often obscure due to the complexity of human development. The human genome contains approximately 25,000 genes and most of them become active to build both tissue and body structures (Brunner and van Driel, 2004). Moreover, growth and morphogenesis of the human embryo relies on the precise orchestration and intercalation of multiple cellular functions, and the spatio/temporal control of the inherent molecular and biological processes. Therefore, modern human genetics regards the detailed understanding of genes and molecular strategies involved as "an indispensable investment" that can foster greater progress in the diagnosis and treatment of these human disorders.

From the beginning of the last century, going back to the Spemann and Mangold experiments, cell to cell signalling has been recognized as one fundamental principle of animal development (Freeman and Gurdon, 2002). At almost every developmental stage cells communicate with each other and such processes permit the generation of cell-type differences during development and the coordination of cell functions during tissue/organ morphogenesis or tissue/organ homeostasis (Freeman and Gurdon, 2002; Pires-daSilva and Sommer, 2003).

Chemical communication is by far the major form of information transfer between cells. Following release by instructive cells, signals move towards target cells through either direct contact or by short and long diffusion (Freeman and Gurdon, 2002; Papin et al., 2005). On target cells signals are captured by distinct cellular receptors that upon integrating and interpreting them activate appropriate intracellular signalling pathways and effectors to modify cell fate, metabolism or function (Freeman and Gurdon, 2002; Pires-daSilva and Sommer, 2003).

Research in the past two decades has yielded important advances towards the identification of the signal proteins, receptors, and intracellular proteins involved in signalling processes. For example the human genome contains more than 1500 genes that encode receptor proteins, and the number of different receptor proteins is further increased by alternative RNA splicing and post-translational modifications. Surprisingly, genetic and biochemical studies revealed that only a few different classes of signalling pathways mediate patterning of a wide variety of cells, tissues and organs. For example, Fibroblast growth factors (FGF) Hedgehog (Hh), Wingless related (Wnt), Transforming growth factor-b (TGF-b) and Notch are used reiteratively during development to mediate very different biological processes in different animals (Freeman and Gurdon, 2002; Pires-daSilva and Sommer, 2003). In other words, a signal that in one instance will cause a cell to differentiate terminally will elsewhere lead another cell type to undergo mitosis and in a third context will trigger cell death.

These findings have raised the question of how generic signals can trigger tissue-specific responses. As a general principle specificity relies on the repertoire of receptors and intracellular mediators that are active in a given cell at a given time (Freeman and Gurdon, 2002). Nevertheless, there is now clear evidence that specificity of signal outcome is also the product of biological strategies ensuring signal level, strength, duration and its spatio-temporal distribution (Freeman and Gurdon, 2002). For example, several of these signalling molecules function as morphogens that form concentration gradients across developmental fields and specify different cell fates in a concentration dependent fashion during pattern formation (Freeman and Gurdon, 2002). Other studies have also shown that differences in the kinetics of the ligand or receptor binding mode, and changes in the temporal and quantitative supply of active ligand can contribute to increases in the heterogeneity of biological responses to incoming signals, but without losing the cell specific effects that ensure reproducibility of developmental processes (Freeman and Gurdon, 2002).

In the pursuit of molecular mechanisms that underlie these further layers of regulation attention has progressively shifted towards components of the extracellular matrix. Besides being structural scaffolds, these proteins are now evaluated as vital elements of the cell signalling machinery that provide processing and bioavalaibility of instructive signals (Bernfield et al., 1999; Bulow and Hobert, 2006).

In particular, cell surface proteoglycans such as Glypicans (Gpcs) interact with chemokines, growth factors/morphogens and their receptors (Bulow and Hobert, 2006; Hacker et al., 2005; Nybakken and Perrimon, 2002). Disruption of Gpc functions in *Drosophila*, Zebrafish, *Xenopus Laevis* and mouse results in phenotypes reminiscent of defects in cellular responses to regulatory signalling molecules (Hacker et al., 2005; Lin, 2004). Yet, genetic and embryological studies link Gpcs to the regulation of cell signalling events during morphogenesis and adult physiology (Bishop et al., 2007; DeBaun et al., 2001; Hacker et al., 2005; Lin et al., 1999). In humans, mutations in the *Gpc-3* gene are associated with several diseases. For example, mutations in the *Gpc-3* gene underlie a condition called Simpson-Golabi-Behmel syndrome, which is characterized by overgrowth of the body and other birth defects (DeBaun et al., 2001). Homozygosity for null mutations in the *Gpc-6* gene cause autosomal recessive omodysplasia, a genetic condition characterized by severe short stature and congenital heart defects (Campos-Xavier et al., 2009). Additionally, increased and decreased activity of some *Gpcs* (including *Gpc*-1, -3, -4 and -6) occurs in certain forms of cancer (Filmus, 2001). Here, we review our current knowledge on the implication of these proteoglycans in congenital malformations, and discuss our understanding of their mechanism of action.

2. Molecular design of cell surface glypicans

The name "glypicans" identifies a family of heparan sulphate proteoglycans (HSPGs) that are linked to the exocytoplasmic surface of the plasma membrane through a covalent glycosyl-phosphatidylinositol (GPI) linkage (Bulow and Hobert, 2006). Together with Syndecans, *gpc* gene products are the major cell surface HSPGs (Bulow and Hobert, 2006). Gpcs have been highly conserved throughout evolution and most likely arose early during metazoan evolution (Filmus et al., 2008). In this section, we describe their major structural features that have been crucial to elucidate their in vivo roles.

2.1 Glypican assembly

Gpcs are proteins of around 60–70 kDa with a characteristic pattern of 14-conserved cysteine residues mainly located to the central domain (De Cat and David, 2001). Gpcs also share an N-terminal signal sequence and a hydrophobic C-terminal sequence involved in the formation of the GPI anchor structure (Fig. 1; De Cat and David, 2001). Heparan sulphate glycosaminoglycan (HSGAG) polysaccharide side chains can be attached to serine residues in consensus sequences, such as XGlyXGlySerX, that are located between the central domain and the C-terminal GPI-anchor (De Cat and David, 2001). The HSGAG of proteoglycans can undergo complex patterns of modification consisting of sulphations of hydroxyl groups in individual sugar molecules, epimerizations of specific carbon atoms and changes in length of the individual sugar residues (Bulow and Hobert, 2006; Nybakken and Perrimon, 2002). Such modifications are thought to generate a large structural diversity that might encode information for the selective binding of protein ligands (Bulow and Hobert, 2006; Nybakken and Perrimon, 2002). In general, Gpcs carry these HS chains, but Gpc5 also displays chondroitin sulfate modifications (Saunders et al., 1997).

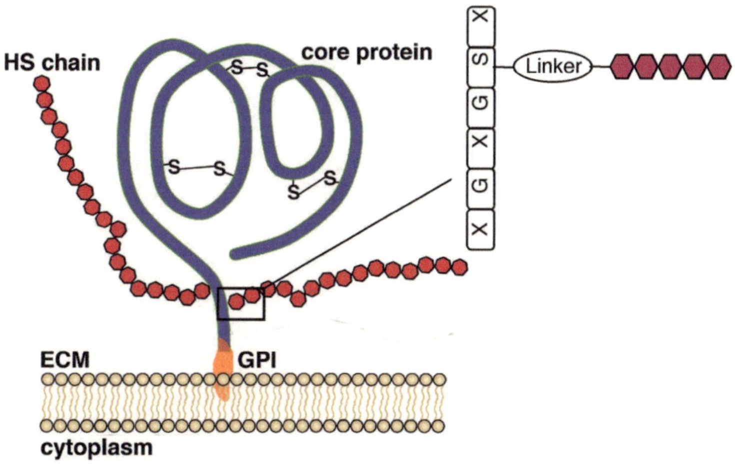

Fig. 1. Schematic representation of the Gpc structure.

The glypican core protein spans the extracellular space. Disulfide bridge (S-S) are thought to organize the core protein as a compact globular domain. HS chains are covalently bound to serine residues that are part of X-Gly-X-Gly-Ser-X motifs in the polypeptide chain close to the plasma membrane. The carboxyterminus of Gpcs is covalently linked to the plasma membrane via a GPI anchor. Red filled hexagon chains represent HS chains. S = serine; G = glycine; X = aminoacid (adapted from De Cat, B. and David, G., 2001).

Proteolytic cleavages of the core proteins can also contribute to generate distinct Gpc forms. As shown for several vertebrate and invertebrate proteins, the N-terminal cysteine-rich domain of Gpcs can be splitted from the HS-modified and GPI-anchored C-terminal domain following endo-proteolytic processing (Song and Filmus, 2002). To which extent this event occurs in physiological condition is matter of investigation because the ratio between uncleaved and cleaved Gpcs varies according to the *gpc* family member and the tissue-specific context. The N-terminal Gpc fragment is not membrane-associated and, once generated, it can remains linked to its C-terminal half through one or more disulfide bridges (De Cat et al., 2003; Eugster et al., 2007). Thus, proteolytic processing can provide a molecular strategy to rapidly make available a secreted Gpc product, if needed, as such a form could be released from producing cells simply following redox changes of the extra-cellular environment.

2.2 Evolutionary origins

Gpcs are evolutionarily conserved proteins found in organisms as distinct as nematodes, fruit flies and mammals (De Cat and David, 2001; Fico et al., 2007; Filmus et al., 2008). The human and mouse genome contain six Gpc family members, *Gpc-1* to *Gpc-6* in humans and *gpc-1* to *gpc-6* in mice (De Cat and David, 2001; Fico et al., 2007; Filmus et al., 2008) whereas five *gpc*-like genes have been identified in zebrafish (Filmus et al., 2008; Topczewski et al., 2001), two in *Drosophila* (*dally* and *dally-like*; Baeg et al., 2001; Nakato et al., 1995) and two in *C. elegans* (*gpn-1* and *lon-2*; Gumienny et al., 2007; Hudson et al., 2006). The amino acid sequences of mammalian Gpc vary from being 17% to 63% identical. However, sequence relationships and exon organizations suggest that mammalian *gpcs* consist of two distinct subfamilies (De Cat and David, 2001; Fico et al., 2007; Filmus et al., 2008). The first subfamily includes *gpc*-1, -2, -4 and -6 genes with amino acid sequence homology ranging from 40–60% and composed of nine exons. The other subfamily incorporates *gpc*-3 and -5, with amino acid sequences 40% identical and containing eight exons. Of note, *gpc*-6 maps near to *gpc*-5 on mouse chromosome 14 and on human chromosome 13. *Gpc*-4, which is most homologous to *gpc*-6 maps to chromosome Xq26 near to *gpc*-3, which is highly related to *gpc*-5 (De Cat and David, 2001; Fico et al., 2007; Filmus et al., 2008). Therefore, members of the different subfamilies are inclined to cluster on the same chromosome. Whether *gpc* subfamilies and the genomic linkage of different members have evolved from a series of gene and genome duplications is still a matter of debate. In support of this possibility there are studies in organisms such as *Drosophila* and zebrafish showing the existence of distinct orthologs for each mammalian subfamily and their genomic linkage (Filmus and Capurro, 2008). It will be interesting to examine to what extent the appearance of *gpc* subfamilies might underlie the evolution of functional similarities in members of the same subfamily and functional differences among those more divergent. In this context, studies on *Dally* and *Dally-like* aimed at distinguish their activity on Hh have shown that *Dally-like* but not *Dally* is required for Hh response in a *Drosophila* cultured cell assay (Williams et al., 2010). Intriguingly, Gpc-4 and -6, which are the mammalian Gpcs most closely related to *Dally-like*, complement *Dally-like* function in this biological system (Williams et al., 2010). In contrast, *Dally* and its ortholog Gpc-3 exhibit trans-dominant negative activities (Williams et al., 2010). These studies suggest a large trend in which related Gpc members may have evolved similar activities in distinct cellular contexts, but further understanding will come from studies on other signalling activities.

3. Glypicans: From structural compounds to signalling molecules

Once considered as acting merely as structural components of the extra cellular matrix, Gpcs are now widely recognized as essential modulator of many biological processes. These include their role as carriers in cellular uptake of growth promoting polyamines such as spermine (Casero and Marton, 2007; Fransson et al., 2004). It has been proposed that the binding of Gpcs to polyamines is mediated by electrostatic interactions occurring between Gpc HS side chains and polyamine residues. After transport to endosomes, HS moieties are degraded by nitric oxide. This is expected to weaken HS interaction with polyamines and results in their unloading and possibly exit from endosomes to elicit functions. The mechanisms underlying polyamines uptake has been analyzed in several systems and discussed in previous reports (Belting, 2003; Fransson et al., 2004).

To date, Gpcs are also considered as potential carriers of cell-penetrating peptides. Cell-penetrating peptides are short cationic peptides extensively studied in medicine as drug delivery agents for the treatment of different diseases including cancer and virus infection (Rajendran et al. , 2010). Their entry into cells is typically initiated through interaction with cell-surface HS proteoglycans (HSPGs) via electrostatic interactions, followed by endocytosis (Poon and Gariepy, 2007). Studies on the intracellular delivery of cell-penetrating peptides have shown that the migration of these peptides into cells as well as their final destination could depend on the nature of the HSPGs expressed at the cell surface (Poon and Gariepy, 2007). The GPI-anchor typical of Gpc proteins provides them with specific membrane-trafficking properties distinct from those of transmembrane HS molecules such as Syndencans (Chatterjee and Mayor, 2001; Payne et al., 2007). Therefore, Gpcs mediated uptake of cell-penetrating peptide is currently evaluated as a new strategy to enhance target-specific delivery of a large variety of entrapped therapeutic drugs.

Research on Gpcs has further increased due to the discovery that they act at the interface between the extra cellular environment and the inner cellular domain to fine tune inputs triggered by key secreted regulatory proteins. Although Gpcs have important physiological roles (Bishop et al., 2007), we concentrate here on their developmental functions and on the molecular mechanisms by which Gpcs trigger cell fate and tissue pattern.

3.1 Glypicans as modulator of regulatory extra-cellular signals

Our knowledge of Gpc biology has significantly expanded over the past decade with the discovery that Gpcs are not simply structural proteins. Being mostly extracellular, Gpcs are involved in the regulation of various signalling pathways triggered by secreted peptides including that of Wnt, Fgf, Hh, bone morphogenic protein (Bmp), insulin-like growth factor and hepatocyte growth factor (Fico et al., 2007; Filmus and Capurro, 2008).

The functional relevance of Gpcs as signalling modulators has come from the genetic analysis and embryological manipulation of Gpcs in different species and in cultured cells (Table 1).

Core protein	Species	Major defect	Affected Signals	References
Lon-2	*C elegans*	Body length	Bmp	Gumienny TL, Curr Biol 2007
Dally	Drosophila mutant	Embryogenic epidermis	Hg, Wg	Nybakken K, Biochim Biophys Acta 2002 Han C, Development 2004
		Wing imaginal discs	Hg, Wg	Nybakken K, Biochim Biophys Acta 2002 Han C, Development 2004
		Eye-antennal discs	Dpp	Hacker U, Nat Rev Mol Cell Biol 2005 Lin X, Development 2004
		Germline stem cells	Bmp	Guo Z, Development 2009
Dally-like	Drosophila mutant	Wing imaginal disc	Wg	Nybakken K, Biochim Biophys Acta 2002 Kreuger J, Dev Cell 2004 Kirkpatrick CA, Dev Cell 2004
		Tracheal morphogenesis	Fgf	Yan D, Dev Biol 2007
Knypek	Zebrafish mutant	Gastrulation	Wnt	Topczewski J, Dev Cell 2010; Caneparo L, Genes Dev 2007; Sepich DS, Development 2011
		Cartilage/ bone morphogenesis	Wnt	LeClair EE, Dev Dyn 2009
gpc4	Xenopus morpholino	Gastrulation Dorsal forebrain	Wnt Fgf	Song HH, J Biol Chem 2005 Galli A, Development 2003
gpc1	Mouse null allele	Early neurogenesis	Fgf	Jen YH, Neural Dev 2009
gpc3	Mouse null allele	Body size	Wnt	Song HH, J Biol Chem 2005
		Limb mesenchyme	Bmp	Grisaru S, Dev Biol 2001
		Ureteric mesenchyme	Bmp, Fgf	Paine-Saunders S, Dev Biol 2000

Table 1. Glypicans function in model organisms. This table reports the major phenotypes observed by genetic and embryological studies on *glypican* genes and the main involved signals

For example, in vitro studies have shown that Gpc4 positively modulated hepatocyte growth factor activity during renal epithelial branching morphogenesis (Karihaloo et al., 2004). Mice lacking Gpc3 are affected by overgrowth, renal cystic dysplasia and limb defects. Some of these phenotypes are consistent with defects in Wnt and Bmp signalling pathways, respectively (Grisaru et al., 2001; Paine-Saunders et al., 2000; Song et al., 2005). Additional studies have also shown that the developmental overgrowth observed in *gpc3*-null mice is, at least in part, a consequence of the hyperactivation of the Hh pathway indicating that Gpc3 inhibits Hh (Gallet et al., 2008; Capurro et al., 2009). Interestingly, Gpc5 stimulates the proliferation of rhabdomyosarcoma cells by eliciting a positive action on Hh signalling (Li et al., 2011), in contrast to the Gpc3-mediated negative control of Hh.

These findings reveal that members of the Gpc family can display opposite roles in the regulation of a given signalling protein. The *C. elegans* Gpc Lon-2 also controls body size length (Gumienny et al., 2007). It has been proposed that Lon-2 negatively regulates Bmp signalling as *lon-2* mutants recapitulate phenotypes caused by Bmp over-expression (Gumienny et al., 2007). Another example is the Zebrafish *knypek*, which encodes the *gpc* homolog to mammalian Gpc4/Gpc6 (Topczewski et al., 2001). *knypek* controls convergent-extension movements during zebrafish gastrulation by positively modulating Wnt11 activity (Topczewski et al., 2001).

Modulation of extra-cellular signals by Gpcs has also been reported in *Xenopus*. In particular, reducing Gpc4 (Xgly4) disrupts cell movements during gastrularion (Ohkawara et al., 2003). We have also shown that loss-of Gpc4 function in *Xenopus* embryos impairs forebrain patterning and cell survival from early neural plate stages onwards, and that these early developmental defects result in brains affected by microcephaly at later stages (Fig. 2; Galli et al., 2003). Xgly4 physically interacts with Wnt11, and might enhance function in the Wnt/PCP pathway during gastrulation (Ohkawara et al., 2003). In addition to Wnt11, we have demonstrated that Xgly4 also binds Fgf2. Inhibition of Fgf signalling results in dorsal forebrain phenotypes similar to those of Xgly4 depleted embryos, indicating that establishment and patterning of the dorsal forebrain territory may require modulation of Fgf signalling by Xgly4 (Galli et al., 2003).

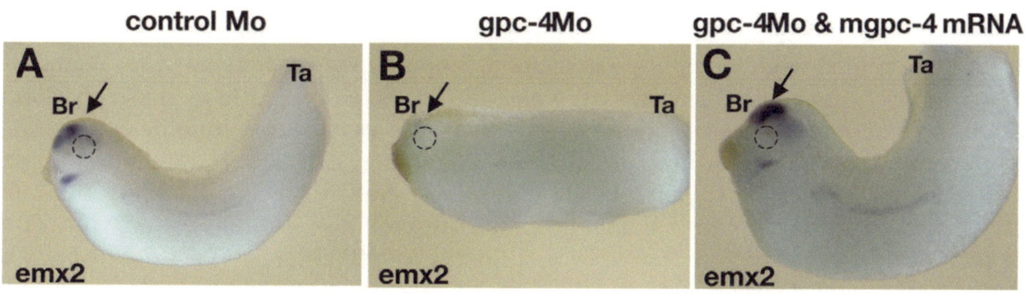

Fig. 2. Forebrain defects in GPC-4 depleted embryos. Side view of Xenopus embryos at tail bud stage showing expression of the dorsal forebrain marker *emx-2* as detected by whole mount in situ hybridization (arrow in all panels). Xenopus embryos were injected at 2 cell stage with morpholino oligos to interfere with Gpc-4 activity. Injections were done by using control morpholino (*control*Mo), or morpholino targeting *gpc-4* (*gpc-4*Mo). Embryos were also co-injected with morpholino targeting *gpc4* (*gpc-4*Mo) and mouse *gpc-4* mRNA (*mgpc-4* mRNA) for rescue experiments. (**A, B**) *emx-2* expression in the dorsal forebrain of tailbud embryos; note the loss of *emx-2* expression and the forebrain microcephalic morphology in GPC-4 depleted embryos (**B**). (**C**) Rescue of *emx-2* expression and forebrain morphology in a tail bud embryo co-injected with Gpc-4Mo and *mGpc-4* mRNA. Br: brain; Ta: Tail.

In *Drosophila* the Gpc *Dally-like* is required for Hh signalling in the embryonic ectoderm whereas both Gpcs *Dally* and *Dally-like* are required and redundant in Hh movement in developing wing imaginal discs (Han et al., 2004; Yan and Lin, 2009). Additional studies on the wing disc patterning have also demonstrated that in *Dally* and *Dally-like* mutants the distribution and signalling of Wnt and Bmp family members, Wingless (Wg) and Decapentaplegic (Dpp) respectively, are altered (Nybakken and Perrimon, 2002).

Furthermore, *Dally* and *Dally-like* also act on Wg during segment polarity determination and on Dpp in the developing eye and antennal discs (Hacker et al., 2005; Lin, 2004). Overall, these and other studies reveal that different cell types can take advantage of Gpc-mediated regulation to control signal supply during distinct developmental processes. In addition, they show that vertebrate and invertebrate Gpcs have diverse and specialized functions towards a given signalling protein including their capability of enhancing or suppressing its activity in a stage- and/or tissue-specific regulated manner.

3.2 Heparan sulphate chains and core proteins for signal control

The findings that Gpcs enable cells controlling activity of a wide range of extracellular effectors with greater selectivity towards biological outcomes, suggest that Gpcs are rather dynamic proteins capable of employing various mechanisms to exert their regulatory effects in biological processes. One question that has arisen is whether these properties are conferred by their unique structural motifs. As discussed above, Gpcs are most likely globular proteins with HS chains at the carboxyl terminus. Of note, Chen and Lander have identified that the Gpc1 globular domain is a structural motif that potently influences HS substitutions (Chen and Lander, 2001). Moreover, it has been proposed that the physical constraint of HS attachment sites at the carboxyl terminus could result in proteins with HS chains in the proximity of the cell surface. These basic structural features, together with the known versatile conformation and orientation of HS functional groups, could prime Gpc HS modifications to a degree that facilitate their contacts with cell-membrane proteins (e.g. signalling receptors) while retaining specificity in binding modes (Tumova et al., 2000). The GPI-anchorage is yet another feature that makes Gpc proteins subject to distinct subcellular localization and intracellular trafficking processes as well as to release into the extracellular environment through shedding mechanisms involving distinct extracellular lipases (Chatterjee and Mayor, 2001; Payne et al., 2007). Gpcs trafficking and shedding can both lead to a gain of signal, down-regulation properties and cell non-autonomous activities (Yan and Lin, 2009). These issues are the subjects of intense investigation, and a growing body of data is being published on Gpc mechanism of action. In this paragraph we briefly summarize the current state of our knowledge related to HS-mediated Gpc activity. We focus more on studies showing that the core protein and its GPI anchor confer on Gpcs additional functional versatility.

3.2.1 The heparan sulphate chains

The hypothesis that functional Gpc properties are mediated by HS modifications was first evaluated for the Fgf/Fgf receptor axis as it is well established that Fgfs rely on the co-receptor role of HSPGs for receptor binding and activation. As demonstrated by experiments performed mainly in cultured cells and in cell-free systems, Gpc HS modifications can catalyze binding of Fgfs to their receptors and boost receptor activation and its biological functions. For example, purified HS chains derived from Gpc-1, following protease-mediated digestion, augment the binding of Fgf-2 and Fgf-1 to Fgf receptor 1 to an extent that lower concentrations of ligands are needed for activation (Bonneh-Barkay et al., 1997b). Also, the Gpc-dependant Fgf binding and activation of receptors is nearly abolished when cells are treated with chlorate to inhibit Gpc sulfatation (Steinfeld et al., 1996). In this context, covalent cross-linking of Fgf-2 to cells expressing its receptor demonstrates a putative Fgf-2/Fgf receptor complex when HS modified Gpcs are present in the same cell (Steinfeld et al., 1996). A conclusion that can be drawn from these studies is that cell-surface Gpcs by means of their HS modification can function as essential partners for the Fgf tyrosine kinase receptor. Potential mechanisms of action may include immobilizing of the ligand, increasing its local concentration, presenting it to a signalling receptor, or otherwise modifying the molecular encounters between ligands and receptors. The expected overall effect is thus enhancing receptor activation at low ligand concentrations. Interestingly, whereas Gpc-1 HS chains potentiate the biological activity of Fgf-1 they strongly inhibit Fgf-7 function (Berman et al., 1999; Bonneh-Barkay et al., 1997a). This suggests that HS chains can also act as a dual modulator of biological activities exerting both stimulatory and inhibitory effects depending on factors involved. More recently, experimental settings involving depletion of these sulphate groups both in vivo and in cultured cells have demonstrated that Gpcs HSs mediate interaction with additional HS binding proteins and impact their activity. This includes the binding and stimulation of Wg (the drosophila homolog of Wnt) signalling in the wing imaginal disc by *Dally* as well as the ability of human Gpc-5 to interact with Hh and enhance its growth promoting activity in rhabdomyosarcoma cells (Yan and Lin, 2009; Li et al. , 2011,). Interestingly, Dally HS chains are required in vivo to activate high-threshold but not low-threshold target genes of Dpp (Kirkpatrick et al., 2006), suggesting that HSPG core proteins could serve distinct functions in low- versus high-threshold morphogenetic signalling.

Recent studies have revealed that the co-receptor function of Gpcs can also provide a new paradigm of cell-cell communication. In the stem cell niche associated with germ cells the Gpc Dally is critical for making and maintaining the female germ cells (Hayashi et al., 2009). However, in this stem cell niche, *dally* is expressed by the cap cells, which also produce the Dpp signalling molecule, but not in the receiving cells (germ cells), which instead express Dpp receptor (Hayashi et al., 2009). These findings have raised questions and interest about the underlying molecular mechanisms. Studies in cultured cells have provided evidence that Dally enhances Dpp signalling in *trans* through a contact-dependent mechanism allowing the complementation of co-receptor-receptor complexes in adjacent cells (Dejima et al., 2011). Therefore, unlike typical co-receptor functions, Dally can serves as a *trans* co-receptor for Dpp when it has to enhance its signalling on neighboring cells. So far the mechanism for contact-dependent signalling has been mainly attributed to membrane-bound ligands and receptors such as Delta-Notch and Ephrins and their receptor tyrosine kinases (Hainaud et al., 2006). The fact that Gpcs act as *trans* activator partners establishes new strategies for crosstalk between adjacent cells during tissue assembly and maintenance.

In conclusion, a common theme throughout all studies is that HS chains are responsible for different aspects of Gpc biology. By means of HS chains Gpcs sequester secreted soluble ligands and modulates their activity. As co-receptors and *trans* co-receptor, Gpcs modulate ligand-receptor encounters that can activate and inhibit cell proliferation, motility, and differentiation. Also HS side chains are not uniform and changes in the distribution of sulphate groups may affect ligand-binding properties and biological outcomes in a cell type-specific manner.

3.2.2 The glypican core proteins

The GPI anchor and the core protein are two additional structural motifs that impinge on functional versatility of Gpcs at different levels. Most insights have come from cell biological approaches undertaken to investigate how Gpcs affect Hh and Wg signalling and gradient formation.

Concerning Wg, genetic analysis of Dally-like in the wing imaginal discs has highlighted a role for this Gpc in polarizing the Wg morphogenetic gradient. In the wing imaginal disc, Wg is secreted by a narrow strip of cells located at the dorsal–ventral boundary and spreads over a distance of up to 20 cell diameters. Wg first accumulates on the cell surface apical side in expressing cells to be then re-distributed to the basolateral membrane of receiving cells, where it is released in association with lipoprotein particles (Panakova et al., 2005; Strigini and Cohen, 2000). It has been proposed that polarizing Wg on the cell membrane allows the subsequent polarization of morphogen distribution within an epithelium, thus resulting in distinct tissue patterns (Marois et al., 2006). Therefore, one major question in the field is how Wg reaches the basolateral cell surface when it is secreted apically. Gallet and colleagues have investigated the subcellular localization of Dally-like in this cellular system and shown that Dally-like, which is apically targeted by means of its GPI anchor, undergoes internalization and redistribution to the basolateral membrane through a dynamin-dependent endocytosis (transcytosis; Fig. 3; Gallet et al., 2008). Interestingly, Wg is no longer detected at the basolateral surface of cells away from the Wg source in mutant cells lacking Dally-like protein. Moreover, tethering Dally-like at the cell membrane (by replacing the GPI anchor with a trans-membrane domain) strongly stabilized Wg at the apical surface while decreasing the amount of Wg at the basolateral compartment (Gallet et al., 2008). Altogether, these findings support the view that Wg is secreted apically and it is then endocytosed with the help of Dally-like (Fig. 3). Once internalized, Dally-like targets Wg by transcytosis to the basolateral compartment, where it is stabilized and can then spread farther away in a polarized manner (Fig. 3); Gallet et al., 2008). These findings also open the intriguing possibility that Dally-like-mediated basolateral polarization of Wg accounts for Wg activity in long-range signalling (Gallet et al., 2008). However, whether this mechanism underlies distinct Wg signalling activity remains a matter of debate (Williams et al.; Yan et al., 2009).

In contrast to the Wg situation, GPI-mediated endocytosis of Gpcs appears directly implicated in modulating Hh signalling in a positive and negative manner. For example, Dally-like endocytosis from the cell surface catalyzes the internalization of Hh in flies. In this context, internalization of Hh occurs together with its receptor Patched (Fig. 4; Gallet et al., 2008). Removing Patched from the membrane alleviates the inhibition of the transmembrane protein Smoothened by Patched and enables Smoothened to activate Hh target genes (Fig. 4; Gallet et al., 2008). Complementary studies performed in mice have revealed that the mammalian Gpc-3, via its GPI-anchor, also mediates internalization of Shh (the vertebrate homolog of Hedgehog) and regulates its signalling, with however opposing outcomes. Indeed, through endocytosis Gpc-3 inhibits Shh activity rather than activating it as in flies (Fig. 4; Capurro et al., 2008; Gallet et al., 2008). It has been proposed that Gpc-3 has high affinity for Shh and can, therefore, compete with Patched for Shh binding (Capurro et al., 2008). Upon binding, Gpc-3 targets Shh to endocytic vesicles for degradation, thus leaving the unliganded Ptc at the cell surface, and free to inhibit Smoothened (Fig. 4; Capurro et al., 2008). This possibility is also consistent with results showing that hyperactivation of Shh can in part explain the Simpson-Golabi-Behmel overgrowth syndrome caused by loss-of-function mutations in Gpc-3, and with other experiments revealing an increased expression of Shh target genes in Gpc-3 deficient mice and mouse embryonic fibroblasts (Capurro et al., 2008).

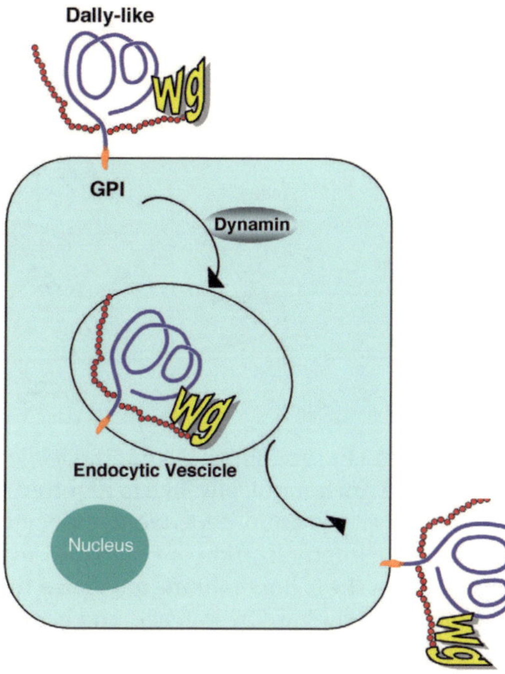

Fig. 3. The GPI anchor of Dally-like triggers Wg transcytosis. The GPI anchor of Dally-like is required for its apical targeting, subsequent internalization through dynamin-dependent endocytosis and relocalization to the basolateral compartment. It has been proposed that Wg is secreted apically and is then endocytosed with the help of Dally-like. Once internalized, Dally-like targets by transcytosis Wg to the basolateral compartment , where it is stabilized and can then spread farther away in a polarized manner (adapted from Dong Yan and Xinhua Lin 2008).

Interestingly, the Gpc3 core protein (without HS chains) binds with high affinity to Shh in cultured cells independently of its HS chains, while it does not interact with Patched (Capurro et al., 2008). These findings raise the possibility that the Gpc core protein cooperate with the GPI motif to establish differences in Gpc binding properties of signalling molecules, which will in turn affect biological readout. Of note, Williams and colleagues found that the Dally-like core protein without HS chains substantially rescues lack of Hh signalling in Dally-like mutant embryos, demonstrating specific activity for this structural domain (Williams et al., 2010). Similarly, the core proteins of the mammalian Gpc-4 and -6, which are the closest relatives of Dally-like, allow full dose-dependent re-activation of Hh, in contrast to Gpc-2, -3 and -5 that have no activity (Williams et al., 2010). This configuration of sequence homology and functional conservation suggests that the two major Gpc subfamilies have evolved similar roles in Hh signalling control (see also above). Therefore, Gpc agonistic and antagonistic signalling activities should also be identifiable in the Gpc core protein.

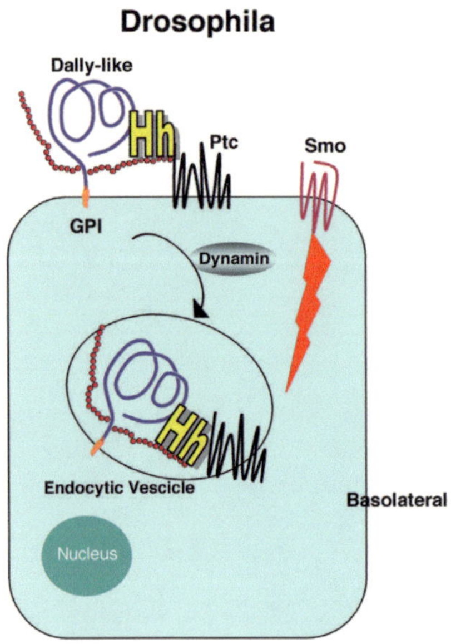

Fig. 4. Opposing roles for Gpcs in Hh signalling. (**A**) In *Drosophila* wing discs, Dally-like promotes Hh signalling. The GPI anchor of Dally-like is required for its apical targeting and subsequent internalization through dynamin-dependent endocytosis. Dally-like endocytosis from the cell surface catalyzes the internalization of Hh in flies that occurs together with Patched (Ptc). Removing Ptc from the cell membrane alleviates the inhibition of the transmembrane protein Smoothened (Smo) by Patched and enables Smoothened to activate Hh target genes. (**B**) In mouse development, Gpc3 acts as an inhibitor of Hh signalling. The Gpc3 core binds Shh on the cell surface and compete with Patched for Shh binding. Upon binding, Gpc-3 targets Shh to endocytic vesicles for degradation, thus leaving the unliganded Ptc at the cell surface, and free to inhibit Smoothened (adapted from Dong Yan and Xinhua Lin 2008).

To date, additional studies support the idea that the protein cores selectively impact on functions of distinct Gpcs. For example, as opposed to the positive role of Dally in Wg signalling (Lin and Perrimon, 1999), Dally-like shows biphasic activities: as repressor for Wg short-range signalling and as activator for long-range responsiveness. It has been proposed that the Dally-like core protein has high binding affinity for Wg (Yan et al., 2009), a property that allows Dally-like to bind and retain Wingless on the cell surface. Interestingly, ectopic expression of Dally-like inhibits activation of Wg targets. In contrast, increasing the expression of the Wg receptor Frizzled leads to their activation (Yan et al., 2009). These and other results suggest that the physiological role of Wg is linked to the cellular ratio between Dally-like and Frizzled (Yan et al., 2009). In other words, Dally-like binds and retains Wingless on the cell surface away from its receptor Frizzled. However, Dally-like can also facilitate Wg binding to Frizzled depending on the ratio of ligand, receptor and Dally-like. Although intriguing, these results arise additional question that need to be answered. For example, how different is the affinity of Dally and Dally-like core proteins for Wg? Do Dally-like related mammalian Gpcs show dual roles in Wg modulation? Is there any specific protein domain required for Wg binding? Concerning the latter question, it has been proposed that Wg binding could occur via the N-terminal domain of Dally-like (Yan et al., 2009).

Moreover, structural analysis combined with structure-guided mutagenesis also suggests that this domain could guide Dally-like/Shh interaction (Kim et al., 2011). Further studies will address whether and in which manner the N-terminal domain impacts Gpc activity.

In conclusion, the studies above discussed begin to unravel how Gpcs fulfil diverse functions in signalling pathways during development. In particular, they highlight the importance of GPI-mediated Gpc endocytosis in participating at the control of Wingless intracellular trafficking and possibly gradient formation, and in the modulation of Hh signalling in different biological context. Other important findings are the demonstration that Gpcs core proteins show binding affinity for certain signals independent of HS-side chains, and that they can modulate events as opposed as signal activation and inhibition. Thus, core proteins of Gpcs appear to ensure on its own an additional degree of signal modulation that increases specificity of biological readouts.

4. Glypicans in human diseases

Genome-wide linkage scan and mutation analysis have revealed that alteration in GPC functions can underlie human congenital malformation compromising developmental events such as bone growth and heart pattern formation. This discovery has permitted a better comprehension of pathophysiology of these disorders, their diagnosis and management. The generation of animal models has significantly broadened the understanding of these distinct developmental processes and their molecular bases.

4.1 The Simpson-Golabi-Behmel Syndrome

The Simpson-Golabi-Behmel Syndrome is an X-linked overgrowth disorder characterized by pre- and postnatal overgrowth, minor facial anomalies, skeletal defects, polydactyly and fingernail hypoplasia, small bulge in the small intestine, umbilical or inguinal hernia, genitourinary abnormalities, heart defects, supernumerary nipples and an increased risk of neonatal death (Gurrieri et al. , 2011). In patients there is also an increased risk of embryonal tumour development, mainly Wilms' tumour. Mental retardation is not constantly found and is usually mild (Gurrieri et al. , 2011).

Pilia and colleagues uncovered the genetic bases of this disorder in 1996 with the demonstration that mutations in the *Gpc-3* gene are responsible for a large proportion of Simpson-Golabi-Behmel Syndrome cases. Since then, different *Gpc-3* mutations have been identified in patients and these were found to be rather heterogeneous ranging from large chromosomal rearrangements to micro deletions and point mutations in different exons (Gurrieri et al. , 2011; Hughes-Benzie et al., 1996; Pilia et al., 1996; Sakazume et al., 2007; Xuan et al., 1999). Sequence analysis of mutated loci, led to the proposal that Simpson-Golabi-Behmel Syndrome is caused by a non-functional GPC-3 protein while additional unknown genetic factors were possibly responsible for the phenotypic variations among patients. The role of GPC-3 in this disorder was then confirmed by the generation of *Gpc-3*-deficient mice, since these mice recapitulate several phenotypes of the Simpson-Golabi-Behmel Syndrome patients including developmental outgrowth and dysplastic kidneys (Cano-Gauci et al., 1999; Paine-Saunders et al., 2000). Moreover, recent findings showing that GPC3 polymorphisms have a significant impact in the body size of mice have provided additional support for a role of GPC3 in the regulation of body size (Oliver et al., 2005).

At a cellular level the tissue overgrowth syndrome of *Gpc-3*-deficient mice appears to be a consequence of an increased proliferation rate, which is consistent with the possibility that Gpc-3 acts as a negative regulator of cell proliferation in the mouse embryo (Hartwig et al., 2005). However, Gpc-3 can also induce apoptosis in a cell-type specific manner suggesting that enhanced cell survival may also contribute to the overgrowth defects (Filmus, 2001), Interestingly, Simpson-Golabi-Behmel Syndrome patients develop embryonal tumours (see above). Moreover, *Gpc-3* expression is markedly decreased in human gastric cancer. Therefore, it is likely that in humans Gpc-3 functions also as a tumour suppressor gene (Gonzalez et al., 1998).

One of the current major challenges is to identify the GPC-3 targets relevant for the pathogenesis of this complex disease. It has been proposed that GPC-3 inhibits embryonic growth by negatively regulating Insulin-like growth factor-II (Pilia et al., 1996). However, studies in cultured cells have failed to detect any biochemical or genetic interaction between Gpc-3 and the Insulin-like growth factor-II signalling pathway (Cano-Gauci et al., 1999; Chiao et al., 2002; Song et al., 2005). Capurro and colleagues explored the possibility that Gpc-3 acts as a negative regulator of body size by inhibiting two mammalian Hh proteins: Shh and Indian Hh (see also above; Capurro et al., 2008; Capurro et al., 2009). The rational behind this approach is linked to findings revealing that 1) these two Hh family members are both present in the developing embryo, with Shh more widely expressed and Indian Hh restricted to the developing bones; 2) hyperactivation of the Hh signalling pathway in mice causes overgrowth phenotypes (Makino et al., 2001; Milenkovic et al., 1999); 3) in humans, Patched mutations are linked to Gorlin's Syndrome, a disorder causing multiple basocellular carcinomas accompanied by large head size, longer-larger bones, and polydactyly (Hahn et al., 1996). As discussed above, secreted Hh proteins binds and antagonizes the function of the Patched receptor known to block the activity of the signalling effector Smoothened. Binding of Hhs to Patched thus results in the activation of Smoothened, which in turn transduces the Hh signal intracellularly leading to the activation of Hh target genes such as Gli and Patched (Hooper and Scott, 2005). In a first study, Capurro and colleagues compared the degree of activation of the Hh signalling pathway in *gpc-3* null mouse embryos and culture cells as well as potential Gpc-3/Shh protein interaction (Capurro et al., 2008). Results showed that the levels of Shh protein and of its targets increases in structures affected by Simpson-Golabi-Behmel Syndrome (e.g. gut and digits). As discussed above, they also uncovered that Gpc-3 can bind Shh and activate its signalling pathway, and acts as a competitive inhibitor of the Shh-Patched interaction, and triggers Shh endocytosis and degradation (Capurro et al., 2008). Therefore, a reasonable picture that can be drawn from these studies is that Gpc-3 normally restrains Hh signalling to control body size. Lack of Gpc-3 leads to the hyperactivation of this pathway causing the overgrowth phenotype of the Simpson-Golabi-Behmel Syndrome patients (Capurro et al., 2008).

To provide further genetic evidence that the Hh signalling pathway mediates, at least in part, the regulatory activity of Gpc-3 on embryonic growth, Capurro and colleagues performed a second study where they attempted to rescue the overgrowth phenotype of Gpc-3 deficient embryos by crossing them with mice carrying an Indian Hh null allele (Capurro et al., 2009). Indian Hh was chosen because its activity is more confined to endochondral skeleton. Indeed, Indian Hh deficient mice show a severe growth deficiency in the endochondral skeleton as a result of a reduced chondrocyte proliferation and maturation, as well as osteoblast formation (St-Jacques et al., 1999). In contrast, Viviano and colleagues reported an abnormal persistence of hypertrophic chondrocytes in Gpc-3-deficient embryonic bones and a delay in endochondral ossification (Viviano et al., 2005). As for Shh, Gpc-3 deficient mice show more Indian Hh and Patched protein levels in the developing long bones (Capurro et al., 2009). Moreover the overgrowth syndrome of Gpc-3 deficient mice is partially rescued in the Indian Hh null background (Capurro et al., 2009). Therefore, the author proposed that the accumulation of Indian Hh as a result of the lack of Gpc-3 might be the cause of an unbalance rate of chondrocyte proliferation versus differentiation, which ultimately causes the longer bone overgrowth found in mutant mice (Capurro et al., 2009; Viviano et al., 2005). Although further investigations will elucidate how lack of Gpc-3 affects development at the cellular level, these genetic studies provide important clues on the molecular basis of Simpson-Golabi-Behmel Syndrome in humans by beginning to unravel the aberrant signalling mechanisms. Moreover, they have also told us that more broad approaches such as tissue micro-arrays need to be taken into account to understand this complex disorder. In this context, the *gpc-3*-deficient mouse model will be instrumental to identify and evaluate the involvement of other signalling pathways as well as to determine whether Gpc-3 has tissue specific effects in this disease. Of note, there are the studies on the *gpc-3*-deficient mice indicating that an impairment of the Fgf/Shh signalling axis in the embryonic hearts could underlie the congenital cardiac malformations in Simpson-Golabi-Behmel syndrome (St-Jacques et al., 1999) while the renal dysplasia could be linked to an inbalance of stimulatory and inhibitory signals (e.g. Fgf-7 and Bmp-2 respectively) during tissue morphogenesis (Grisaru et al., 2001).

Further help in understanding the involvement of *Gpc-3* in this human disorder could come from attempts to define structural-functional relationships associated with specific *Gpc-3* mutations in humans. Interestingly, one Simpson-Golabi-Behmel Syndrome patient has a deletion affecting both *Gpc-3* and *Gpc-4,* which is found immediately centromeric to *Gpc-3* at Xq26 (Veugelers et al., 1998). Recently, a wide screening has identified patients carrying mutations in the *Gpc-4* but not in the *Gpc-3* gene (Waterson et al., 2010). We anticipate that future research will extensively evaluate whether connections between GPC-4 functions and the clinical features of this syndrome exist.

4.2 Autosomal-recessive omodysplasia

Autosomal recessive omodysplasia is a genetic condition characterized by skeletal and craniofacial defects (Maroteaux et al., 1989). Skeletal abnormalities include shortening and distal tapering of the humerus and femur, proximal radioulnar diastasis, and anterolateral radial head dislocation. In patients with autosomal recessive omodysplasia both upper and lower limbs are affected in contrast to the dominant form of the disorder in which the lower limbs are normal. Facial defects comprise frontal bossing, a flat nasal bridge, low set ears, a long philtrum, anteverted nostrils, and frontal capillary hemangiomas. Variable findings are hernias, congenital heart defects, mental retardation and delayed motor development. Being recessive, autosomal recessive omodysplasia is a rare disorder with an incidence of <1 / 1000000 and, to date, around 22 cases of recessive omodysplasia have been described. Recent advances in understanding its pathophysiology have come from Campos-Xavier and collaborators reporting that the autosomal-recessive omodysplasia maps to chromosome 13

(13q31.1-q32.2; (Campos-Xavier et al., 2009). By performing fine analysis of candidate genes, Campos-Xavier and collaborators have further linked autosomal recessive omodysplasia to point mutations or to larger genomic rearrangements in the *Gpc-6* gene (Campos-Xavier et al., 2009).

All mutations found in the individuals affected by omodysplasia predict absence of a functional protein. Hypothetical mutant proteins would be truncated and thereby lose both the GPI and the HS-binding sites, essential for the putative GPC-6 functions (Campos-Xavier et al., 2009). Similarly to *Gpc-3*, *Gpc-6* mutations are also found in the entire coding region without any mutational hotspot and include one or more exons. Recently, *Gpc-5* haploinsufficiency has been proposed as the molecular cause of upper limb anomalies and growth retardation in 13q deletion syndrome because of its expression in the developing limb (Quelin et al., 2009). *Gpc-5* colocalises with *Gpc-6* on 13q31.2–q31.3, and the two genes are clustered, similarly to *Gpc-3* and *Gpc-4* on chromosome X, suggesting that these members of the *Gpc* family share an evolutionary link (see also above; Filmus, 2001) that might reflect a common function (De Cat and David, 2001; Paine-Saunders et al., 2002; see also above). However, because GPC-5 does not compensate for loss of GPC-6 in omodysplasia patients, their functional relationship is not supported.

Axial bone growth occurs through growth plates in which chondrocytes undergo proliferation, hypertrophy, cell death, and osteoblastic replacement (Ornitz and Marie, 2002). The immature chondrocytes are rapidly proliferating cells characterized by a small size and irregular shape. In the hypertrophic cartilage zone, chondrocytes make matrix and enlarged lacunae. The pathological characteristics of the omodysplastic growth plates are an expanded zone of proliferating cartilage and an increased number of closely packed, small chondrocytes suggesting that omodysplasia is due to an impaired endochondral ossification (Borochowitz et al., 1998). During endochondral ossification, *Gpc-6* is predominanlty expressed in the proliferative zone decreasing dramatically in the prehypertrophic and hypertrophic zones (Campos-Xavier et al., 2009). These expression data correlate with the morphologic findings in the human omodysplasia. They also correlate with the distribution of Indian Hh, Fgf, Bmp and Wnt proteins, which are known to regulate endochondral ossification (Ornitz and Marie, 2002) and to have the potential of functionally interacting with Gpc-6. Moreover, the etiology of many other human skeletal dysplasias with defects in endochondral ossification has been attributed to specific mutations in the gene encoding FGF receptor 3 (Ornitz and Marie, 2002). The international mouse strain resource (IMSR ; http://www.findmice.org/) has recently generated different mouse strains carrying loss of function mutations in the *gpc-6* gene but to our knowledge, no studies have been yet reported. The functional analysis of *gpc-6* mutant mice will be crucial to establish the involvement of Gpc-6 functions in this disorder and to uncover the cellular and molecular basis of all associated clinical features.

5. Conclusion and future direction

Research over the past years has advanced our understanding of Gpc functions during mammalian development and the list of human syndromes associated with their aberrant function is likely to grow. Indeed, recent studies have described *Gpc-5* and *Gpc-6* as candidate genes for postaxial polydactyly type A, an inherited human condition causing digit duplications (van der Zwaag et al. , 2010). Gpc genes have also been linked to other less defined human diseases, such bipolar disorder and Sudden Cardiac Arrest (Arking et al. 2011; Maheshwari et al., 2002) and further studies will clarify their involvement. We and others have shown that Gpcs are among the most abundant HSPGs in the developing nervous system and are expressed in embryonic and adult neural stem cells (Bandtlow and Zimmermann, 2000; Hagihara et al., 2000; Luxardi et al., 2007). Our embryological manipulations in *Xenopus* embryos have begun to provide insight into their role in brain size as abrogation of Gpc4 activity in *Xenopus* embryos disrupts forebrain patterning and cell survival, and causes microcephaly (see also above and Ficure 2; Galli et al., 2003). Therefore, our findings raise the possibility that some of the congenital microcephalies may arise as a consequence of disrupting *Glpc-4* gene function during brain development.

As discussed above, Gpc genes are inclined to cluster on the same chromosome. Simpson-Golabi-Behmel patients can carry deletions that affect not only the *Gpc-3* but also the *Gpc-4* gene. In mouse, *gpc-3* shows distinct expression patterns compared to *gpc-4* and the latter is highly expressed in the developing brain and kidney (Luxardi et al., 2007). Therefore, it is possible that mutation in the *Gpc-4* gene also contribute to aspects of the Simpson-Golabi-Behmel syndrome. Further studies will require the analysis of *gpc* compound mutant embryos and mice as they could recapitulates additional clinical features of this syndrome.

A second major area of research will concern the identification of the pathological signalling events underlying the clinical features of disorders associated with abnormal GPC functions. When analysing pathologies involving GPC, it is important to take into account that these diseases might be also linked to GPC gain-of-functions rather then loss-of-functions. The gene targeting approach in mice has begun to clarify this issue. As described above, Gpcs control different signalling proteins in a cell-type and developmental-stage specific manner. Therefore, further studies will require tissue- and stage-specific loss-of-function mutations of *gpc* genes. We think that a better understanding of Gpc involvement in normal and pathological processes, as well as the identification of the associated signals can hopefully provide a wider clinical spectrum for the development of targeted therapies.

6. Acknowledgment

We thank Keith Dudley for critically reading the manuscript, Flavio Maina for helpful discussions, and Antonella Galli for contributing to Figure 2. This work was supported by the Marie Curie Host Grant for TOK (MTKD-CT-2004-509804), by the FRM (n° DLC20060206414) and by AFM (n° 13683).

7. References

Arking, D.E., Reinier, K., Post, W., Jui, J., Hilton, G., O'Connor, A., Prineas, R.J., Boerwinkle, E., Psaty, B.M., Tomaselli, G.F., Rea, T., Sotoodehnia, N., Siscovick, D.S., Burke, G.L., Marban, E., Spooner, P.M., Chakravarti, A. and Chugh, S.S. (2011) Genome-wide association study identifies GPC5 as a novel genetic locus protective against sudden cardiac arrest. *PLoS One*, 5, e9879.

Baeg, G.H., Lin, X., Khare, N., Baumgartner, S. and Perrimon, N. (2001) Heparan sulfate proteoglycans are critical for the organization of the extracellular distribution of Wingless. *Development*, 128, 87-94.

Bandtlow, C.E. and Zimmermann, D.R. (2000) Proteoglycans in the developing brain: new conceptual insights for old proteins. *Physiol Rev*, 80, 1267-1290.

Belting, M. (2003) Heparan sulfate proteoglycan as a plasma membrane carrier. *Trends Biochem Sci*, 28, 145-151.

Berman, B., Ostrovsky, O., Shlissel, M., Lang, T., Regan, D., Vlodavsky, I., Ishai-Michaeli, R. and Ron, D. (1999) Similarities and differences between the effects of heparin and glypican-1 on the bioactivity of acidic fibroblast growth factor and the keratinocyte growth factor. *J Biol Chem*, 274, 36132-36138.

Bernfield, M., Gotte, M., Park, P.W., Reizes, O., Fitzgerald, M.L., Lincecum, J. and Zako, M. (1999) Functions of cell surface heparan sulfate proteoglycans. *Annu Rev Biochem*, 68, 729-777.

Bishop, J.R., Schuksz, M. and Esko, J.D. (2007) Heparan sulphate proteoglycans fine-tune mammalian physiology. *Nature*, 446, 1030-1037.

Bonneh-Barkay, D., Shlissel, M., Berman, B., Shaoul, E., Admon, A., Vlodavsky, I., Carey, D.J., Asundi, V.K., Reich-Slotky, R. and Ron, D. (1997a) Identification of glypican as a dual modulator of the biological activity of fibroblast growth factors. *J Biol Chem*, 272, 12415-12421.

Bonneh-Barkay, D., Shlissel, M., Berman, B., Shaoul, E., Admon, A., Vlodavsky, I., Carey, D.J., Asundi, V.K., Reich-Slotky, R. and Ron, D. (1997b) Identification of glypican as a dual modulator of the biological activity of fibroblast growth factors. *J Biol Chem*, 272, 12415-12421.

Borochowitz, Z., Sabo, E., Misselevitch, I. and Boss, J.H. (1998) Autosomal-recessive omodysplasia: prenatal diagnosis and histomorphometric assessment of the physeal plates of the long bones. *Am J Med Genet*, 76, 238-244.

Brunner, H.G. and van Driel, M.A. (2004) From syndrome families to functional genomics. *Nat Rev Genet*, 5, 545-551.

Bulow, H.E. and Hobert, O. (2006) The molecular diversity of glycosaminoglycans shapes animal development. *Annu Rev Cell Dev Biol*, 22, 375-407.

Campos-Xavier, A.B., Martinet, D., Bateman, J., Belluoccio, D., Rowley, L., Tan, T.Y., Baxova, A., Gustavson, K.H., Borochowitz, Z.U., Innes, A.M., Unger, S., Beckmann, J.S., Mittaz, L., Ballhausen, D., Superti-Furga, A., Savarirayan, R. and Bonafe, L. (2009) Mutations in the heparan-sulfate proteoglycan glypican 6 (GPC6) impair endochondral ossification and cause recessive omodysplasia. *Am J Hum Genet*, 84, 760-770.

Cano-Gauci, D.F., Song, H.H., Yang, H., McKerlie, C., Choo, B., Shi, W., Pullano, R., Piscione, T.D., Grisaru, S., Soon, S., Sedlackova, L., Tanswell, A.K., Mak, T.W., Yeger, H., Lockwood, G.A., Rosenblum, N.D. and Filmus, J. (1999) Glypican-3-deficient mice exhibit developmental overgrowth and some of the abnormalities typical of Simpson-Golabi-Behmel syndrome. *J Cell Biol*, 146, 255-264.

Capurro, M.I., Xu, P., Shi, W., Li, F., Jia, A. and Filmus, J. (2008) Glypican-3 inhibits Hedgehog signaling during development by competing with patched for Hedgehog binding. *Dev Cell*, 14, 700-711.

Capurro, M.I., Li, F. and Filmus, J. (2009) Overgrowth of a mouse model of Simpson-Golabi-Behmel syndrome is partly mediated by Indian hedgehog. *EMBO Rep*, 10, 901-907.

Casero, R.A., Jr. and Marton, L.J. (2007) Targeting polyamine metabolism and function in cancer and other hyperproliferative diseases. *Nat Rev Drug Discov*, 6, 373-390.

Chatterjee, S. and Mayor, S. (2001) The GPI-anchor and protein sorting. *Cell Mol Life Sci*, 58, 1969-1987.

Chen, R.L. and Lander, A.D. (2001) Mechanisms underlying preferential assembly of heparan sulfate on glypican-1. *J Biol Chem*, 276, 7507-7517.

Chiao, E., Fisher, P., Crisponi, L., Deiana, M., Dragatsis, I., Schlessinger, D., Pilia, G. and Efstratiadis, A. (2002) Overgrowth of a mouse model of the Simpson-Golabi-Behmel syndrome is independent of IGF signaling. *Dev Biol*, 243, 185-206.

De Cat, B. and David, G. (2001) Developmental roles of the glypicans. *Semin Cell Dev Biol*, 12, 117-125.

De Cat, B., Muyldermans, S.Y., Coomans, C., Degeest, G., Vanderschueren, B., Creemers, J., Biemar, F., Peers, B. and David, G. (2003) Processing by proprotein convertases is required for glypican-3 modulation of cell survival, Wnt signaling, and gastrulation movements. *J Cell Biol*, 163, 625-635.

DeBaun, M.R., Ess, J. and Saunders, S. (2001) Simpson Golabi Behmel syndrome: progress toward understanding the molecular basis for overgrowth, malformation, and cancer predisposition. *Mol Genet Metab*, 72, 279-286.

Dejima, K., Kanai, M.I., Akiyama, T., Levings, D.C. and Nakato, H. (2011) Novel contact-dependent bone morphogenetic protein (BMP) signaling mediated by heparan sulfate proteoglycans. *J Biol Chem*, 286, 17103-17111.

Eugster, C., Panakova, D., Mahmoud, A. and Eaton, S. (2007) Lipoprotein-heparan sulfate interactions in the Hh pathway. *Dev Cell*, 13, 57-71.

Fico, A., Maina, F. and Dono, R. (2007) Fine-tuning of cell signaling by glypicans. *Cell Mol Life Sci*, 68, 923-929.

Filmus, J. (2001) Glypicans in growth control and cancer. *Glycobiology*, 11, 19R-23R.

Filmus, J. and Capurro, M. (2008) The role of glypican-3 in the regulation of body size and cancer. *Cell Cycle*, 7, 2787-2790.

Filmus, J., Capurro, M. and Rast, J. (2008) Glypicans. *Genome Biol*, 9, 224.

Fransson, L.A., Belting, M., Cheng, F., Jonsson, M., Mani, K. and Sandgren, S. (2004) Novel aspects of glypican glycobiology. *Cell Mol Life Sci*, 61, 1016-1024.

Freeman, M. and Gurdon, J.B. (2002) Regulatory principles of developmental signaling. *Annu Rev Cell Dev Biol*, 18, 515-539.

Gallet, A., Staccini-Lavenant, L. and Therond, P.P. (2008) Cellular trafficking of the glypican Dally-like is required for full-strength Hedgehog signaling and wingless transcytosis. *Dev Cell*, 14, 712-725.

Galli, A., Roure, A., Zeller, R. and Dono, R. (2003) Glypican 4 modulates FGF signalling and regulates dorsoventral forebrain patterning in Xenopus embryos. *Development*, 130, 4919-4929.

Gonzalez, A.D., Kaya, M., Shi, W., Song, H., Testa, J.R., Penn, L.Z. and Filmus, J. (1998) OCI-5/GPC3, a glypican encoded by a gene that is mutated in the Simpson-Golabi-Behmel overgrowth syndrome, induces apoptosis in a cell line-specific manner. *J Cell Biol*, 141, 1407-1414.

Grisaru, S., Cano-Gauci, D., Tee, J., Filmus, J. and Rosenblum, N.D. (2001) Glypican-3 modulates BMP- and FGF-mediated effects during renal branching morphogenesis. *Dev Biol*, 231, 31-46.

Gumienny, T.L., MacNeil, L.T., Wang, H., de Bono, M., Wrana, J.L. and Padgett, R.W. (2007) Glypican LON-2 is a conserved negative regulator of BMP-like signaling in Caenorhabditis elegans. *Curr Biol*, 17, 159-164.

Gurrieri, F., Pomponi, M.G., Pietrobono, R., Lucci-Cordisco, E., Silvestri, E., Storniello, G. and Neri, G. (2011) The Simpson-Golabi-Behmel syndrome: A clinical case and a detective story. *Am J Med Genet A*.

Hacker, U., Nybakken, K. and Perrimon, N. (2005) Heparan sulphate proteoglycans: the sweet side of development. *Nat Rev Mol Cell Biol*, 6, 530-541.

Hagihara, K., Watanabe, K., Chun, J. and Yamaguchi, Y. (2000) Glypican-4 is an FGF2-binding heparan sulfate proteoglycan expressed in neural precursor cells. *Dev Dyn*, 219, 353-367.

Hahn, H., Wicking, C., Zaphiropoulous, P.G., Gailani, M.R., Shanley, S., Chidambaram, A., Vorechovsky, I., Holmberg, E., Unden, A.B., Gillies, S., Negus, K., Smyth, I., Pressman, C., Leffell, D.J., Gerrard, B., Goldstein, A.M., Dean, M., Toftgard, R., Chenevix-Trench, G., Wainwright, B. and Bale, A.E. (1996) Mutations of the human homolog of Drosophila patched in the nevoid basal cell carcinoma syndrome. *Cell*, 85, 841-851.

Hainaud, P., Contreres, J.O., Villemain, A., Liu, L.X., Plouet, J., Tobelem, G. and Dupuy, E. (2006) The role of the vascular endothelial growth factor-Delta-like 4 ligand/Notch4-ephrin B2 cascade in tumor vessel remodeling and endothelial cell functions. *Cancer Res*, 66, 8501-8510.

Han, C., Belenkaya, T.Y., Wang, B. and Lin, X. (2004) Drosophila glypicans control the cell-to-cell movement of Hedgehog by a dynamin-independent process. *Development*, 131, 601-611.

Hartwig, S., Hu, M.C., Cella, C., Piscione, T., Filmus, J. and Rosenblum, N.D. (2005) Glypican-3 modulates inhibitory Bmp2-Smad signaling to control renal development in vivo. *Mech Dev*, 122, 928-938.

Hayashi, Y., Kobayashi, S. and Nakato, H. (2009) Drosophila glypicans regulate the germline stem cell niche. *J Cell Biol*, 187, 473-480.

Hooper, J.E. and Scott, M.P. (2005) Communicating with Hedgehogs. *Nat Rev Mol Cell Biol*, 6, 306-317.

Hudson, M.L., Kinnunen, T., Cinar, H.N. and Chisholm, A.D. (2006) C. elegans Kallmann syndrome protein KAL-1 interacts with syndecan and glypican to regulate neuronal cell migrations. *Dev Biol*, 294, 352-365.

Hughes-Benzie, R.M., Pilia, G., Xuan, J.Y., Hunter, A.G., Chen, E., Golabi, M., Hurst, J.A., Kobori, J., Marymee, K., Pagon, R.A., Punnett, H.H., Schelley, S., Tolmie, J.L., Wohlferd, M.M., Grossman, T., Schlessinger, D. and MacKenzie, A.E. (1996) Simpson-Golabi-Behmel syndrome: genotype/phenotype analysis of 18 affected males from 7 unrelated families. *Am J Med Genet*, 66, 227-234.

Karihaloo, A., Kale, S., Rosenblum, N.D. and Cantley, L.G. (2004) Hepatocyte growth factor-mediated renal epithelial branching morphogenesis is regulated by glypican-4 expression. *Mol Cell Biol*, 24, 8745-8752.

Kim, M.S., Saunders, A.M., Hamaoka, B.Y., Beachy, P.A. and Leahy, D.J. (2011) Structure of the protein core of the glypican Dally-like and localization of a region important for hedgehog signaling. *Proc Natl Acad Sci U S A*, 108, 13112-13117.

Kirkpatrick, C.A., Knox, S.M., Staatz, W.D., Fox, B., Lercher, D.M. and Selleck, S.B. (2006) The function of a Drosophila glypican does not depend entirely on heparan sulfate modification. *Dev Biol*, 300, 570-582.

Li, F., Shi, W., Capurro, M. and Filmus, J. (2011) Glypican-5 stimulates rhabdomyosarcoma cell proliferation by activating Hedgehog signaling. *J Cell Biol*, 192, 691-704.

Lin, X., Buff, E.M., Perrimon, N. and Michelson, A.M. (1999) Heparan sulfate proteoglycans are essential for FGF receptor signaling during Drosophila embryonic development. *Development*, 126, 3715-3723.

Lin, X. and Perrimon, N. (1999) Dally cooperates with Drosophila Frizzled 2 to transduce Wingless signalling. *Nature*, 400, 281-284.

Lin, X. (2004) Functions of heparan sulfate proteoglycans in cell signaling during development. *Development*, 131, 6009-6021.

Luxardi, G., Galli, A., Forlani, S., Lawson, K., Maina, F. and Dono, R. (2007) Glypicans are differentially expressed during patterning and neurogenesis of early mouse brain. *Biochem Biophys Res Commun*, 352, 55-60.

Maheshwari, M., Christian, S.L., Liu, C., Badner, J.A., Detera-Wadleigh, S., Gershon, E.S. and Gibbs, R.A. (2002) Mutation screening of two candidate genes from 13q32 in families affected with Bipolar disorder: human peptide transporter (SLC15A1) and human glypican5 (GPC5). *BMC Genomics*, 3, 30.

Makino, S., Masuya, H., Ishijima, J., Yada, Y. and Shiroishi, T. (2001) A spontaneous mouse mutation, mesenchymal dysplasia (mes), is caused by a deletion of the most C-terminal cytoplasmic domain of patched (ptc). *Dev Biol*, 239, 95-106.

Marois, E., Mahmoud, A. and Eaton, S. (2006) The endocytic pathway and formation of the Wingless morphogen gradient. *Development*, 133, 307-317.

Maroteaux, P., Sauvegrain, J., Chrispin, A. and Farriaux, J.P. (1989) Omodysplasia. *Am J Med Genet*, 32, 371-375.

Milenkovic, L., Goodrich, L.V., Higgins, K.M. and Scott, M.P. (1999) Mouse patched1 controls body size determination and limb patterning. *Development*, 126, 4431-4440.

Nakato, H., Futch, T.A. and Selleck, S.B. (1995) The division abnormally delayed (dally) gene: a putative integral membrane proteoglycan required for cell division patterning during postembryonic development of the nervous system in Drosophila. *Development*, 121, 3687-3702.

Nybakken, K. and Perrimon, N. (2002) Heparan sulfate proteoglycan modulation of developmental signaling in Drosophila. *Biochim Biophys Acta*, 1573, 280-291.

Ohkawara, B., Yamamoto, T.S., Tada, M. and Ueno, N. (2003) Role of glypican 4 in the regulation of convergent extension movements during gastrulation in *Xenopus laevis*. *Development*, 130, 2129-2138.

Oliver, F., Christians, J.K., Liu, X., Rhind, S., Verma, V., Davison, C., Brown, S.D., Denny, P. and Keightley, P.D. (2005) Regulatory variation at glypican-3 underlies a major growth QTL in mice. *PLoS Biol*, 3, e135.

Ornitz, D.M. and Marie, P.J. (2002) FGF signaling pathways in endochondral and intramembranous bone development and human genetic disease. *Genes Dev*, 16, 1446-1465.

Paine-Saunders, S., Viviano, B.L., Economides, A.N. and Saunders, S. (2002) Heparan sulfate proteoglycans retain Noggin at the cell surface: a potential mechanism for shaping bone morphogenetic protein gradients. *J Biol Chem*, 277, 2089-2096.

Paine-Saunders, S., Viviano, B.L., Zupicich, J., Skarnes, W.C. and Saunders, S. (2000) glypican-3 controls cellular responses to Bmp4 in limb patterning and skeletal development. *Dev Biol*, 225, 179-187.

Panakova, D., Sprong, H., Marois, E., Thiele, C. and Eaton, S. (2005) Lipoprotein particles are required for Hedgehog and Wingless signalling. *Nature*, 435, 58-65.

Papin, J.A., Hunter, T., Palsson, B.O. and Subramaniam, S. (2005) Reconstruction of cellular signalling networks and analysis of their properties. *Nat Rev Mol Cell Biol*, 6, 99-111.

Payne, C.K., Jones, S.A., Chen, C. and Zhuang, X. (2007) Internalization and trafficking of cell surface proteoglycans and proteoglycan-binding ligands. *Traffic*, 8, 389-401.

Pilia, G., Hughes-Benzie, R.M., MacKenzie, A., Baybayan, P., Chen, E.Y., Huber, R., Neri, G., Cao, A., Forabosco, A. and Schlessinger, D. (1996) Mutations in GPC3, a glypican gene, cause the Simpson-Golabi-Behmel overgrowth syndrome. *Nat Genet*, 12, 241-247.

Pires-daSilva, A. and Sommer, R.J. (2003) The evolution of signalling pathways in animal development. *Nat Rev Genet*, 4, 39-49.

Poon, G.M. and Gariepy, J. (2007) Cell-surface proteoglycans as molecular portals for cationic peptide and polymer entry into cells. *Biochem Soc Trans*, 35, 788-793.

Quelin, C., Bendavid, C., Dubourg, C., de la Rochebrochard, C., Lucas, J., Henry, C., Jaillard, S., Loget, P., Loeuillet, L., Lacombe, D., Rival, J.M., David, V., Odent, S. and Pasquier, L. (2009) Twelve new patients with 13q deletion syndrome: genotype-phenotype analyses in progress. *Eur J Med Genet*, 52, 41-46.

Rajendran, L., Knolker, H.J. and Simons, K. (2010) Subcellular targeting strategies for drug design and delivery. *Nat Rev Drug Discov*, 9, 29-42.

Sakazume, S., Okamoto, N., Yamamoto, T., Kurosawa, K., Numabe, H., Ohashi, Y., Kako, Y., Nagai, T. and Ohashi, H. (2007) GPC3 mutations in seven patients with Simpson-Golabi-Behmel syndrome. *Am J Med Genet A*, 143A, 1703-1707.

Saunders, S., Paine-Saunders, S. and Lander, A.D. (1997) Expression of the cell surface proteoglycan glypican-5 is developmentally regulated in kidney, limb, and brain. *Dev Biol*, 190, 78-93.

Song, H.H. and Filmus, J. (2002) The role of glypicans in mammalian development. *Biochim Biophys Acta*, 1573, 241-246.

Song, H.H., Shi, W., Xiang, Y.Y. and Filmus, J. (2005) The loss of glypican-3 induces alterations in Wnt signaling. *J Biol Chem*, 280, 2116-2125.

St-Jacques, B., Hammerschmidt, M. and McMahon, A.P. (1999) Indian hedgehog signaling regulates proliferation and differentiation of chondrocytes and is essential for bone formation. *Genes Dev*, 13, 2072-2086.

Steinfeld, R., Van Den Berghe, H. and David, G. (1996) Stimulation of fibroblast growth factor receptor-1 occupancy and signaling by cell surface-associated syndecans and glypican. *J Cell Biol*, 133, 405-416.

Strigini, M. and Cohen, S.M. (2000) Wingless gradient formation in the Drosophila wing. *Curr Biol*, 10, 293-300.

Topczewski, J., Sepich, D.S., Myers, D.C., Walker, C., Amores, A., Lele, Z., Hammerschmidt, M., Postlethwait, J. and Solnica-Krezel, L. (2001) The zebrafish glypican knypek controls cell polarity during gastrulation movements of convergent extension. *Dev Cell*, 1, 251-264.

Tumova, S., Woods, A. and Couchman, J.R. (2000) Heparan sulfate chains from glypican and syndecans bind the Hep II domain of fibronectin similarly despite minor structural differences. *J Biol Chem*, 275, 9410-9417.

van der Zwaag, P.A., Dijkhuizen, T., Gerssen-Schoorl, K.B., Colijn, A.W., Broens, P.M., Flapper, B.C. and van Ravenswaaij-Arts, C.M. (2010) An interstitial duplication of chromosome 13q31.3q32.1 further delineates the critical region for postaxial polydactyly type A2. *Eur J Med Genet*, 53, 45-49.

Veugelers, M., Vermeesch, J., Watanabe, K., Yamaguchi, Y., Marynen, P. and David, G. (1998) GPC4, the gene for human K-glypican, flanks GPC3 on xq26: deletion of the GPC3-GPC4 gene cluster in one family with Simpson-Golabi-Behmel syndrome. *Genomics*, 53, 1-11.

Viviano, B.L., Silverstein, L., Pflederer, C., Paine-Saunders, S., Mills, K. and Saunders, S. (2005) Altered hematopoiesis in glypican-3-deficient mice results in decreased osteoclast differentiation and a delay in endochondral ossification. *Dev Biol*, 282, 152-162.

Waterson, J., Stockley, T.L., Segal, S. and Golabi, M. (2010) Novel duplication in glypican-4 as an apparent cause of Simpson-Golabi-Behmel syndrome. *Am J Med Genet A*, 152A, 3179-3181.

Williams, E.H., Pappano, W.N., Saunders, A.M., Kim, M.S., Leahy, D.J. and Beachy, P.A. (2010) Dally-like core protein and its mammalian homologues mediate stimulatory and inhibitory effects on Hedgehog signal response. *Proc Natl Acad Sci U S A*, 107, 5869-5874.

Xuan, J.Y., Hughes-Benzie, R.M. and MacKenzie, A.E. (1999) A small interstitial deletion in the GPC3 gene causes Simpson-Golabi-Behmel syndrome in a Dutch-Canadian family. *J Med Genet*, 36, 57-58.

Yan, D. and Lin, X. (2009) Shaping morphogen gradients by proteoglycans. *Cold Spring Harb Perspect Biol*, 1, a002493.

Yan, D., Wu, Y., Feng, Y., Lin, S.C. and Lin, X. (2009) The core protein of glypican Dally-like determines its biphasic activity in wingless morphogen signaling. *Dev Cell*, 17, 470-481.

3

Central Nervous System Vascular Malformations

Andrew S. Davidson and Marcus A. Stoodley
Neurosurgery Unit, Australian School of Advanced Medicine, Macquarie University, Sydney, Australia

1. Introduction

A detailed understanding of vascular anatomy and embryology is essential to facilitate appropriate decision-making by clinicians responsible for treating vascular malformations of the central nervous system. The development of the cerebral vasculature has been extensively described in the original works of Streeter [1, 2] and Padgett [3-5], and summarized by Davidson and Morgan [6].

1.1 Development of the cerebral arterial system

With the growth of the developing embryonic brain, increasing requirements for oxygen and metabolic substrates demand a more comprehensive and complex vascular system. Covering the entire neuraxis is a primitive network of mesenchymal cells known as the meninx primitiva. The meninx follows the folds that appear during development of the brain, filling the interhemispheric fissure that forms between the two lateral telencephalic bulges to ultimately become the falx cerebri. At this early stage (embryo < 4 mm length), there is no differentiation into arteries and veins; the irregular network of endothelial vascular channels constitutes a primitive germinal bed of endothelium rather than a true circulatory system. The meninx primitiva differentiates into three discreet layers, which will ultimately become the dura mater, the arachnoid, and the pia mater [7]. Ultimately, angioblastic cells from the meninx become applied to the superficial surface of the developing brain, then penetrate the surface and extend perpendicularly to the pial surface between the glial elements, forming an extensive capillary-like network of endothelial cells (endothelial "buds") [2, 7-9].

Vascular buds ultimately coalesce into larger vascular channels, with afferent channels forming arteries and efferent channels forming veins. On the pial surface of the brain, arterial vessels rise above those that become venous, and where these vessel cross, the artery crosses the vein at approximately right angles. Islands of endothelial cells proliferating within the outer layer of the meninx will eventually coalesce to form the dural venous sinuses; those within the middle layer will develop into the major veins that link the cortex to the dural venous sinuses, and the vessels that ultimately supply and drain the brain parenchyma develop from the inner layer [2].

The primitive internal carotid artery (ICA) develops mainly from the third aortic arch (although minor contributions are made from the first and second arches as well). During the early stages of brain development, the ICA supplies most of the blood to the entire brain through several named branches including the trigeminal, hypoglossal, otic, and the proatlantal intersegmental arteries. These primitive branches are usually transient, although rarely they persist in adults.

Next, two parallel collections of primitive arterial arcades appear along the lateral aspect of the rhombencephalon. These longitudinal neural arteries are supplied from the ICA via the trigeminal arteries, and from what will become the posterior circulation via the developing cervical intersegmental arteries. Ultimately, most of these vascular communications recede, with the fused portion of the longitudinal neural arteries forming the midline basilar artery, and the posterior communicating artery replacing the tentorial artery as the source of collateral supply between the anterior and posterior circulation.

Later, the cervical intersegmental arteries develop into the paired vertebral arteries, and the anterior cerebral artery, anterior choroidal artery and middle cerebral artery arise from the ICA. An arterial plexus develops deep within the anterior interhemispheric fissure, which will later become the anterior communicating artery. Through a series of arterial anastomoses and regressions, the primitive dorsal and ventral ophthalmic arteries evolve into the adult form of the ophthalmic artery. Further evolution of the middle cerebral artery occurs, with hemispheric branches and choroidal arteries developing further, and the posterior cerebral artery arises from the ICA.

Finally, the major components of the arterial Circle of Willis near completion, with the posterior cerebral artery taking up the majority of its supply from the posterior circulation, leaving the posterior communicating artery as an embryological remnant in the majority of cases. The development of the cerebellar arteries occurs later, corresponding to the delayed development of the cerebellum compared to the cerebrum.

1.2 Development of the cerebral venous system

At about the 4 mm stage of embryonic development, a primordial venous channel develops within the meninx primitiva, called the vena capitis medialis. This carries no flow, and merely represents proliferative endothelial cells. The vena capitis medialis quickly disappears, and in its place the vena capitis lateralis, or primitive head sinus, forms. The primitive head sinus develops into three separate dural venous plexuses - anterior (telencephalic, diencephalic, and mesencephalic), middle (metencephalic), and posterior (myelencephalic). The primitive maxillary vein joins the primitive head sinus as its only direct tributary, which drains the optic vesicle.

In subsequent stages, the anterior, middle and posterior plexuses of the primitive head sinus unite to become the adult transverse and sigmoid sinuses [7]. The inferior portion of the primitive head sinus later migrates laterally to become the internal jugular vein, whilst the cranial portion of the sinus ultimately becomes the cavernous sinus.

As the telencephalii develop and expand, expansion of the anterior dural venous plexus occurs, and it is the medial aspects of these expansions that fuse to form the primitive marginal sinus, which fuses with its contralateral counterpart to form the early superior sagittal sinus. This is the dominant venous structure anteriorly, and with further development it progressively incorporates more posterior portions of the dural venous sinuses.

With deepening of the interhemispheric fissure, and lateral evagination of the telencephalic-diencephalic sulcus, the choroidal fissures form. The meninx primitiva, primitive choroid, and arterial supply are drawn into the fissure, which drains via the median prosencephalic vein [7]. With the development of the basal ganglia, primitive internal cerebral veins form and fuse in the midline to form the vein of Galen and straight sinus, replacing the median prosencephalic vein as the main venous drainage of the choroid plexus. The caudal remnant of the median prosencephalic vein becomes part of the vein of Galen complex. Persistence of the median prosencephalic vein is a common finding in vein of Galen malformations. The presence of a persistent falcine sinus (which normally regresses as the straight sinus develops) is also indicative of the arrested venous development that commonly occurs in the setting of a vein of Galen malformation [10].

As the developing cerebral and cerebellar hemispheres expand, the dorsal meninges at the junction of the prosencephalon and mesencephalon remain relatively fixed, forming the tentorial edge. The plexus of veins within the leaves of the tentorium and the tentorial sinus (located medially within the tentorium) persist until after birth [8]. The expanding cerebral hemispheres exert more of an influence on the orientation of the tentorium than the cerebellum, and the tentorium changes from its initial vertical orientation to a more horizontal alignment, causing the transverse sinus to alter its vertical alignment to a more horizontal direction.

Development of emissary veins occurs during the latter stages of venous development. Elongation of the primary pial vein during development of the diencephalon and telencephalon produces the basal vein of Rosenthal, which secondarily becomes connected to the internal cerebral vein [7]. Elongation of the numerous subarachnoid veins that bridge from pia to dura during enlargement of the cerebral hemispheres results in the superficial anastomotic veins, including the vein of Trollard and the vein of Labbé. The middle cerebral vein assumes its adult form only after closure of the Sylvian fissure, and remains separate from the cavernous sinus until after birth [8]. The presence of arteriovenous malformations (AVMs) with venous drainage into the Sylvian veins and cavernous sinus suggests that these malformations develop post-natally.

Although the arterial system is well formed by the end of the embryonic period, the venous system continues to evolve until late in fetal development, with some important changes to the developing venous system occurring after birth.

2. Arteriovenous malformations

2.1 Theories of pathogenesis

AVMs have traditionally been considered congenital lesions, occurring as a result of disordered development of the primordial vasculature in a process described by Yaşargil as a 'proliferative capillaropathy' [11]. This hypothesis has become enshrined as neurosurgical doctrine, even in the absence of any strong evidence to support the theory.

As early as 1984, doubts had arisen regarding the congenital nature of AVMs. Warkany and Lemire recognized that AVMs *"are generally considered congenital, although patients usually are adults 20 to 60 years of age and few have signs or symptoms that go back to early life"*. They acknowledge that AVMs *"are puzzling to teratologists because they occur sporadically and are unassociated with congenital malformations outside the central nervous system"*, and point out *"the unsatisfactory state of our understanding of these malformations ... and recommend them to teratologists for further study"* [12]. In his 1996 paper on the embryological basis of AVMs, Mullan noted that the *"theories of origin are not susceptible to experimental proof and should be accepted or rejected on the basis of the available evidence"* [8].

Conflicting evidence exists regarding the pathophysiology of brain AVMs, with reports of clinical cases supportive of both post-natal development and an embryologic origin [6]. A study examining the difference between birth-to-diagnosis and diagnosis-to-hemorrhage timelines in over 1500 cases suggested that a biological change occurs around 10 years from birth that influences hemorrhage rates in patients with AVMs. The authors concluded that the AVM either was not present before age 10 years, or was present but was biologically inactive prior to this stage [13].

As further research is undertaken exploring the molecular biology of AVMs, evidence is accumulating in support of the alternative hypothesis - that AVMs are an acquired abnormality, developing in the postnatal period. Although an initiating event has yet to be defined, possible candidates include trauma, tissue hypoxia, venous hypertension, infection, inflammation, irradiation, or compression [14, 15]. The primary vascular defect may be the development of a simple arteriovenous fistula [16], with altered hemodynamic stresses occurring in the affected vessels. Further pro-angiogenic vascular remodeling and secondary vascular changes would occur secondary to the hemodynamic stress, producing the characteristic AVM seen in clinical practice [17].

2.2 Genetics

Relatively few cases of familial occurrence of AVM have been reported [18], and genome-wide linkage studies in twins have failed to identify a genetic locus for inherited AVM [19]. Although familial cases can occur, AVMs typically occur in a sporadic fashion [20].

One exception to this rule is the development of multiple AVMs in patients with hereditary hemorrhagic telangiectasia (HHT, or Rendu-Osler-Weber syndrome). HHT is an autosomal dominant disorder producing vascular malformations in multiple organs [21]. Small mucocutaneous telangiectasias typically occur in the oral cavity, nose, conjunctivae, and on the fingertips; AVMs occur in the lung (50% of HHT patients), liver (30%), brain (10%), and spine (1%) [22]. HHT patients represent a very small subset of patients with AVMs (approximately 2% of all AVM patients) [23, 24].

HHT usually results from mutations in the Endoglin (HHT1) gene, or ACVRL1 (HHT2) gene; other less common subtypes include HHT in association with juvenile polyposis (JPHT), HHT3, and HHT4. All of the genes responsible for HHT are involved in the transforming growth factor (TGR-β) superfamily signaling pathway, and mutations result in the development of abnormal vascular structures [22].

The prevalence of AVMs in the population is approximately 0.01% [25]. The estimated prevalence of AVMs in the population of patients with HHT is approximately 5-10% [26], although this may be an under-representation because of the controversy surrounding screening of asymptomatic patients for brain AVMs [22]. In one study where screening was performed in 268 of 1291 HHT patients, 15% of HHT1 patients and 1% of HHT2 patients harbored AVMs [21].

There is an increased risk of multiple AVMs in HHT patients [27]. AVMs in HHT patients do not follow the typical pattern of sporadic AVMs; they can grow or regress, and can recur after angiographically confirmed complete resection [28].

Other developmental syndromes associated with brain AVMs include Wyburn-Mason syndrome and Sturge-Weber syndrome [29-31]. The pathogenesis of these developmental abnormalities is poorly understood, and provides little insight into the molecular biology of sporadic AVMs.

Several studies have examined gene expression in AVMs using gene microarray techniques, with hundreds to thousands of genes of interest reported. In one study, where over 1700 differentially expressed genes were identified, the majority belonged to angiogenesis, vascular matrix, or apoptosis pathways [32]. Significantly upregulated genes include those coding for Ang-2, VEGF-A, the VEGF receptor (Flt1), Integrin αv, Endoglin, MMP-9, and Ephrin-A1; significantly downregulated genes include Krit1, Ang-1, Tie, Tek, Laminin α3, Smoothelin, and Connexin 37 [32-35]. Conflicting gene microarray results have been obtained for CD31 (PECAM-1), with one study demonstrating upregulation, and another demonstrating downregulation [32, 34].

Gene single nucleotide polymorphisms (SNPs) have also been studied in groups of patients with AVMs, with a view to identifying potential genes that may be of prognostic and pathophysiological significance. Polymorphisms in the IL-6, IL-1β, TNF-α, and apolipoprotein-E (ApoE) genes have been associated with increased risk of hemorrhage [36-39], and SNPs in ALK-1 are associated with a susceptibility for AVM formation [15].

2.3 Clinical features

Arteriovenous malformations most commonly present in young patients, with a mean age at diagnosis around 35 years. There does not appear to be a gender predilection. They most commonly present with hemorrhage; many population-based studies and large natural history studies demonstrate that approximately 50% of patients present with AVM rupture [40-51]. The next most common presenting feature is seizure, with 24-36% of patients presenting with generalized or partial seizures. Other reasons for presentation include focal neurologic deficit [52], headache [53-55], or as incidental imaging findings in asymptomatic patients [56, 57].

2.4 Diagnosis, including early detection

Noninvasive imaging modalities including CT, CT angiography, MRI, and MR angiography are extremely valuable in the diagnosis and characterization of brain AVM. Determination of proximity to eloquent structures and accurate measurement of nidal dimensions is important in determining surgical risk. In selected cases, functional MRI [58] and diffusion tensor imaging-based tractography [59] may be useful for providing additional information about the relationship of an AVM to critical neurological structures. Non-enhanced CT and gradient-echo or susceptibility-weighted MRI sequences are particularly useful in demonstrating previous hemorrhage. However, digital subtraction angiograpy remains the gold standard for demonstrating AVM angioarchitecture, and is essential for planning appropriate management strategies [60].

2.5 Treatment

Several options are available for the management of patients with AVMs: microsurgical resection, stereotactic radiosurgery, endovascular treatment, multi-modality treatment, or observation. The preferred management option in each case depends on many factors, including AVM specific factors (such as size, location, arterial and venous anatomy, and mode of presentation), institutional factors (experience of cerebrovascular surgical team, access to stereotactic radiosurgery, availability of endovascular treatment options,), and patient factors (general medical condition, co-morbidities, age, patient preference).

In determining the most appropriate management for an individual patient, the surgeon must balance the risk of intervention with the risk of the natural history and recommend the safest, most efficacious option. Sometimes, the safest option is to do nothing [61]. Ultimately, the risks of management must be acceptable to the patient.

2.6 Prognosis

Without treatment, the overall risk of AVM hemorrhage has been estimated to be 2 to 4.6% per year [40-46]. Previous hemorrhage is a significant risk factor for further hemorrhage; the risk may be as high as 18% in the first year after hemorrhagic presentation [62], returning to baseline within 5 years [63]. Large AVM size, deep and infratentorial location, deep venous drainage, and the presence of associated aneurysms have also been implicated as factors associated with a higher risk of rupture.

Early studies, relying on retrospective audits of hospital charts and taken from the era before modern brain imaging and improvements in intensive care management, reported neurological morbidity and mortality as high as 52-81% following AVM hemorrhage [41, 42, 64]. More recent studies have indicated that the morbidity from AVM hemorrhage is not quite as bad as these figures suggest, with 30-47% of patients suffering a neurologic deficit resulting in a modified Rankin Scale score (mRS) > 1 [44, 65, 66]. Long-term population studies have demonstrated that untreated AVMs are associated with a significant risk of long-term excess mortality that is dramatically reduced but not completely normalized following total excision or occlusion of the AVM [67].

Numerous authors have reported the results of surgical resection. It is generally accepted that the risk of surgery is low (<10%) in Spetzler-Martin (SM) grade 1 and 2 lesions [68-71]. Spetzler-Martin grade 3 AVMs are a heterogenous group, and complication rates depend largely on the morphology of these lesions, with some having a risk profile similar to that of small (SM grade 1 & 2) AVMs, and some having a risk profile similar to that of large (SM grade 4 & 5) AVMs [72-74].

Very few series report the results of surgery for large or giant AVMs. There are many groups who advocate against surgery for SM grade 4 & 5 AVMs because of the perceived high risk of surgery [75]. In those series where surgery was undertaken, even in carefully selected patients, complications occurred in up to 30% [76-81].

Ultimately, each of these sets of published results needs to be taken in context, as the results from different neurosurgical centers will differ as a result of referral patterns, treatment selection biases, and experience of the clinicians. Davidson and Morgan reported the risk of surgery in 640 patient with brain AVM, including an analysis of cases excluded from surgery because of the perceived surgical risk; in this series, the observed risk of adverse outcome related to surgery in SM Grade 1 & 2 patients was 1%, the risk in Grade 3 patients was 14%, and the risk in Grade 4 & 5 patients was 34% [82].

The primary goal of AVM treatment with stereotactic radiosurgery is to obliterate the nidus without the need for operative surgical intervention, removing the risk of future hemorrhage. The efficacy of AVM radiosurgery is much lower than with surgery (obliteration rates range from 36% to 92%, depending on the size of the lesion treated) [83, 84]. Unlike surgery, obliteration is delayed by up to 3 years, and during this time the AVM is still at risk of rupture [85].

There are many reports in the literature relating to the risks of stereotactic radiosurgery, including the risk of rupture during the 'latent interval' between treatment and AVM occlusion. More recent series report hemorrhage after radiosurgery in 3% to 9% of patients [86, 87], radiological imaging changes in up to 46% to 66% (severe in 19%) [84, 88], transient neurological complications in 5% to 17% [89, 90], and permanent neurological complications in 1% to 13% [89, 91].

Complete occlusion of an AVM is rarely achieved with endovascular treatment alone, with most published angiographic cure rates ranging from 16-28% [92-97]. Many of the angiographic cures are in small AVMs, with very few complete occlusions in SM grade 3 AVMs or larger. Even in the most experienced hands, complete occlusion was reported in 51% of patients; however, only 12.5% of patient with SM Grade 3-5 AVMs experienced angiographic cure after Onyx embolization [98]. Combined morbidity and mortality rates in these series range from 5-12%, with more aggressive attempts at complete occlusion generally resulting in higher complication rates [93].

Although multi-modality treatment (incorporating combinations of surgery, embolization, and radiosurgery) appears to be an attractive option for treating these large lesions, cure rates are only in the order of 36% [76], and the cumulative effects of treatment-related morbidity may be much higher than single- or dual-modality management.

2.7 Screening of relatives

There is currently no evidence to support the use of diagnostic imaging to screen for the presence of brain AVMs in asymptomatic patients. However, considerable controversy surrounds the role of screening in HHT patients. Some authors argue that the low risk of hemorrhage combined with the significant risk of treatment does not support the use of screening [22]; others have demonstrated a higher risk of hemorrhage in HHT patients with asymptomatic AVMs, and argue in favor of screening [99]. In these patients, the use of non-invasive imaging (such as MR angiography or contrast-enhanced CT angiography) may be considered.

3. Dural arteriovenous malformations

3.1 Theories of pathogenesis

The earliest discussions of the pathogenesis of dural arteriovenous malformations (DAVMs) focussed on a possible congenital origin [100-103]. Reinforcing this belief is the observation that 3% of DAVMs present before the age of 1 year [104]. The occurrence of DAVMs in the neonatal and pediatric population suggests that congenital factors are at play in at least some of these lesions. Dural sinus malformations almost certainly represent disorders of embryonic venous development [105]; it is unclear whether infantile type DAVMs represent a similar embryological malfunction or reflect a response to intrauterine thrombosis. Adult-type fistulous DAVMs are extremely rare in the pediatric population, representing 0.8% of all pediatric vascular malformations [105]. It is now thought that most of these lesions are acquired in adulthood, and that that congenital DAVMs are exceptionally rare.

Possible precipitating factors such as trauma, tumour, cerebral thrombophlebitis, neurological surgery, or ENT infection, can be demonstrated in 15-32% of cases [106-109]. By including patients with generalised hypercoagulable states (such as peripheral DVT, pregnancy, and use of oral contraceptive pill), a large meta-analysis reported that 66% of DAVMs had some possible predisposing factor [110]. In the remainder, however, no demonstrable precipitant can be identified, and the DAVM is considered to be idiopathic.

Two hypotheses have been proposed in an attempt to explain the development of spontaneous or idiopathic DAVMs. In the first, neovascularization of an organising thrombus within a dural venous sinus is described as the primary event leading to the development of a DAVM [111]. The second theory suggests that some unspecified event (which may be a factor other than venous sinus thrombosis) results in opening of physiological arteriovenous shunts normally located within the dura mater [112, 113].

3.2 Genetics

In contrast to parenchymal AVMs of the brain, which may be congenital lesions, DAVMs are now thought to be acquired. DAVMs have been reported to occur in patients with various systemic conditions, particularly syndromes characterised by connective tissue disorders. Potential associations include: atypical Sturge-Weber related syndrome [114], blue rubber-bleb nevus syndrome [115], congenital toxoplasmosis [116], Ehlers-Danlos syndrome [117-119], fibromuscular dysplasia [117, 120, 121], hereditary hemorrhagic telangiectasia [122, 123], Marfan's syndrome [124], osteogenesis imperfecta [117], polyarteritis nodosa [125], pseudoxanthoma elasticum [126], Rendu-Osler-Weber syndrome [127], syndactyly [128], and von Recklinghausen's disease [129].

These reports are generally isolated to single cases, and whilst an association may be proposed on the basis of sound physiological principles, there is little convincing evidence of a causal relationship.

3.3 Clinical features

The clinical features of DAVMs are almost exclusively related to the pattern of venous drainage. Very few clinical manifestations have been related to arterial phenomena and all of these clinical scenarios can be equally well explained by venous hypertension and congestion causing focal impaired perfusion of neural structures [111, 130]. No angiographic evidence for arterial 'steal' in DAVMs has ever been provided. Orbital venous congestion and hypoxic retinopathy have been proposed as suitable explanations for the common ophthalmological symptoms occasionally attributed to arterial insufficiency [131]. Elevated ocular venous pressures may result in oedema and inflammation in surrounding extra-ocular muscles, causing diplopia unrelated to cranial nerve compression [108].

In most DAVM series, pulsatile tinnitus is the most common complaint, occurring in up to two thirds of patients [132-134]. A bruit is detectable in a variable proportion of patients with subjective tinnitus, with reports ranging from 40% [135] to 96% [136].

In the presence of a DAVM, venous hypertension may occur through one of two mechanisms: increased blood flow through a draining vein, caused directly by arteriovenous shunting; or restricted venous outflow distal to the DAVM (including sinus occlusion) as a result of increased blood flow, elevated pressures, and turbulence in the draining vein [137, 138]. Venous congestion is capable of producing neurological deficits [139], and when this occurs locally, focal neurological deficits occur.

Orbital venous hypertension may result in the 'red-eyed shunt syndrome' [140] or 'dural shunt syndrome' [141]. In the presence of a direct, high flow carotico-cavernous fistula (CCF) the clinical features can occur dramatically; however, with an indirect, low-flow DAVM the patient may be asymptomatic, or gradually develop symptoms that are generally less severe than with a direct CCF [126, 140, 141].

Headache is one of the most common complaints leading to a neurologic assessment [142]; however, patients often present with incidental headache unrelated to their pathology. The headache attributed to DAVM is likely to occur in conjunction with signs of intracranial hypertension due to a decrease in venous outflow or sinus thrombosis [143]. Clinicians must rely on the clinical features of headache to differentiate a clinically significant secondary headache from an unrelated benign headache. These clinical features include: sudden onset of headache; worsening pattern of headache; headache with systemic illness or focal neurological signs and symptoms, including papilledema; headache triggered by cough, exertion, or Valsalva manouver; and headache during pregnancy or post-partum [142].

As opposed to parenchymal AVMs, DAVMs consist of a nidus that is supported by a strong collagenous and fibrous stroma (the dura mater), and as such the nidus of a DAVM is rarely the source of hemorrhage [144]. Accordingly, the presence of retrograde parenchymal venous drainage has been shown to be the primary factor responsible for intracranial hemorrhage in DAVMs. It is the parenchymal veins that traverse the space between the dura and the adjacent brain that are generally the source of intracranial hemorrhage in DAVMs [145]. When these veins fail under hemodynamic stress, intracerebral, subarachnoid, or subdural hemorrhage may occur. Of these anatomical locations, intraparenchymal hemorrhage occurs most commonly [146].

Increased venous pressure at the torcular region can cause headaches, papilledema, and infantile hydrocephalus as a result of global venous hypertension [104]. At the more severe end of the spectrum, global venous hypertension with gross impairment of cerebral venous drainage may result in a more severe, progressive, generalized neurological deficit [147]. Patients may present with an extrapyramidal movement disorder, similar to Parkinson's disease [148, 149]. In extreme cases, patients may present with progressive global cognitive decline, which is often mistakenly diagnosed as Alzheimer's dementia. The dementia occurring as a result of DAVMs presents as a severe, rapidly progressive cognitive decline that resolves following obliteration of the DAVM in most cases.

3.4 Diagnosis

Angiography is the most important diagnostic test in the evaluation of a patient suspected of having a DAVM. Complete 6-vessel cerebral digital subtraction angiography, including assessment of bilateral internal carotid, external carotid, and vertebral arteries is required to confirm the diagnosis, and to adequately define the dural origin of the nidus, the arterial supply, and the pattern of venous drainage. Other imaging modalities may be useful when used in conjunction with angiography.

Standard axial CT images are useful in patients with DAVMs, and are able to complement the angiographic findings by adding information on the following: cerebral abnormalities (including intracranial hemorrhage, cerebral edema, hydrocephalus, infarction, and contrast enhancement of dilated intradural venous structures), osseous abnormalities, and abnormal dural enhancement.

MR imaging plays an important complementary role in the evaluation of DAVMs, particularly in the evaluation of venous congestion, local and regional perfusion, and the assessment of venous sinus thrombosis [150]. It may also permit non-invasive follow-up of treated lesions.

3.5 Treatment

Various management options are available for the management of cranial DAVMs: compression therapy, surgical intervention, endovascular treatment, radiation therapy, or observation. The preferred management option in each case depends on many factors, including DAVM specific factors (such as the location of the DAVM, pattern of venous drainage, number of arterial feeders), institutional factors, and patient specific factors. The natural history of DAVMs with retrograde parenchymal venous drainage suggests that treatment should be considered unless unusual circumstances make the risks of intervention prohibitive. A more conservative approach may be considered in patients with a benign DAVM. The reasons for considering treatment in these patients include progressive neurological deficit (including progressive orbital venous hypertension), or disabling tinnitus.

In a meta-analysis of treatment options, surgery (either alone or in association with pre-operative embolization) was the most effective management option for DAVMs located in the transverse or sigmoid sinus, tentorial incisura, and anterior cranial fossa (ACF) [110]. The small number of cases of superior sagittal sinus (SSS) DAVMs precluded a meaningful statistical analysis; however, the authors also recommended surgical treatment in this group.

With the development of better techniques and materials, the role for endovascular treatments in the management of DAVMs continues to evolve. Endovascular management is often considered the primary treatment option for DAVMs in the cavernous sinus; for DAVMs of the transverse and sigmoid sinus regions, the combination therapy of transarterial embolization and surgery provides a more effective treatment than either treatment alone. Embolization alone may be relatively ineffective in DAVMs of the tentorial incisura, however when used in conjunction with surgery may provide a slight advantage over surgery alone [110]. There is little evidence supporting the use of endovascular treatment in the management of DAVMs of the ACF, SSS, or middle cranial fossa (MCF) location.

One of the greatest problems with transarterial embolization is the high rate of incomplete occlusion due to revascularization of the lesion, particularly if not all feeding vessels have been embolized [151]. The theoretical benefit of transvenous embolization includes a greater likelihood of complete occlusion of the abnormal AV shunts [130]. However, the corollary is that although the transvenous approach may be effective in occluding the site of AV shunting, the draining veins and dural sinuses are thin-walled structures and may be perforated by catheters and guidewires [152].

Although stereotactic radiosurgery is claimed to avoid many of the potential complications of embolization and surgery, it is not completely risk-free. Transient neurological deficits due to treatment occur in up to 10% [153-155], and serious neurological complications have been reported [156]. Questions also remain regarding the long-term efficacy of occlusion following radiosurgery, with recurrences reported after complete angiographic obliteration [157].

3.6 Prognosis

For many years, the location of a DAVM was believed to be an important determinant of its behaviour [158]. Subsequently, more detailed studies have demonstrated that after accounting for the pattern of venous drainage, location has no direct correlation with the behavior or natural history of a particular lesion [106, 107, 134]. Instead, due to local venous anatomy, DAVMs in some locations (such as the ACF and tentorial incisura) are more likely to develop retrograde parenchymal venous drainage; it is this pattern of venous drainage that has been demonstrated to be predictive of aggressive behavior [106, 107, 159-161].

The pattern of venous drainage may be defined according to two commonly used classification systems [106, 107]: Borden type I, or Cognard type I and IIa are benign lesions with no retrograde parenchymal venous drainage; Borden type II and III, or Cognard type IIb, IIa+b, and III-V are aggressive lesions exhibiting various degrees of retrograde parenchymal venous drainage.

The natural history of DAVMs relates to the pattern of venous drainage. In general, the risk of intracranial hemorrhage for all DAVMs is approximately 1.8% per year [132]. However, DAVMs that demonstrate retrograde parenchymal venous drainage are associated with a more aggressive natural history [106, 107, 159, 160]. The risk of intracranial hemorrhage or non-hemorrhagic neurological deficit in DAVMs with retrograde parenchymal venous drainage is 15-30% per year, with an annual risk of death of 10-19% [162, 163]. When intracranial hemorrhage occurs, the effects can be devastating, with a 15-25% risk of death [132, 159, 164], and a 35% risk of rebleeding within 2 weeks if the DAVM remains untreated [164].

Effective treatment of DAVMs, with obliteration of all AV shunting, has been shown to result in reversal of neurological deficits [148, 165-172], including visual loss [173, 174]. However, complications can occur from all modalities of management (including observation alone), and progression of venous thrombosis and venous hypertension resulting in death can occur despite multiple attempts at intervention [175, 176].

Many published series report the initial post-treatment angiogram results as confirmation of angiographic obliteration, without performing delayed angiography. Recurrent DAVM, as well as development of new DAVM at sites remote from the initial lesion, can occur after complete obliteration [177-180]. In view of this finding, some authors recommend angiographic follow-up at least 1 year after treatment, to ensure that long-term occlusion has occurred [179]. Other forms of non-invasive angiography (such as CT or MR angiography) are becoming increasingly useful in the follow-up of these lesions.

3.7 Screening of relatives

There is currently no evidence to support the use of diagnostic imaging to screen for the presence of dural AVMs in asymptomatic patients.

4. Vein of galen malformations

4.1 Theories of pathogenesis

Vein of Galen malformations represent a particular subtype of intracranial vascular malformation, and consist of a single midline venous sac with a direct AV fistula within the wall. True vein of Galen malformations represent an embryonic malformation [181], with the malformation corresponding to the persistent fetal median prosencephalic vein, often in association with other abnormalities of arrested venous development [182]. Aneurysmal dilatation of an embryologically normal vein of Galen due to increased venous drainage from another vascular abnormality within its venous territory does not represent a true vein of Galen malformation. Although this type of aneurysmal dilatation has been classified as a type 4 vein of Galen malformation in the classification system of Yasargil [183], a descriptive term such as secondary vein of Galen aneurysmal dilatation is more informative [182, 184].

The true embryonic form of vein of Galen malformation is different from other pediatric DAVMs [105]. As well as having a different pathogenesis, one of the primary differences between DAVMs and vein of Galen malformations is the primary blood supply of the lesion [185]. In DAVMs the primary blood supply is that of the adjacent dura, whereas in vein of Galen malformations it is that of the adjacent brain parenchyma (arising from the fetal prosencephalic and mesencephalic arterial systems) [181]. Lasjaunias, *et al.* classified pediatric DAVMs into three types [105]: dural sinus malformations, infantile type dural arteriovenous shunts, and adult type dural arteriovenous shunts.

Dural sinus malformations and infantile DAVMs present in neonates and early childhood, and are more likely to represent a congenital abnormality in venous development. The adult type is less frequent, representing less than 1% of all pediatric intracranial AVMs; and when presenting in the pediatric population, tends to occur in older children [105].

4.2 Genetics

At present, the role of genetic factors in the formation of VOGM is unknown. Only 1 case of familial VOGM has been reported [186]. However, mutations in the RASA1 gene have been investigated in association with cutaneous capillary malformation-arteriovenous malformation syndrome, including two patients who also harboured VOGMs [187], raising the possibility that genetic influences may play a role in the development of these malformations.

4.3 Clinical features

Typically, neonates present with severe congestive cardiac failure (CCF), infants present with macrocephaly or hydrocephalus, and older children or adults present with seizures, headaches, or cranial neuropathies resulting from mass effect [186].

4.4 Diagnosis, including early detection

The diagnosis of VOGM is made after detailed clinical examination and investigation. Initial radiological examination includes transfontanel ultrasound and cardiac ultrasound (to assess for associated cardiac abnormalities), and MR Imaging of the brain. Angiography is not recommended in neonates unless urgent endovascular treatment is considered [188].The Bicetre Neonatal Evaluation Score [188] requires evaluation of cardiac, cerebral, respiratory, hepatic, and renal function in order to guide management decisions, and is used to triage neonates to either conservative management, or immediate or delayed endovascular management.

Non-invasive vascular imaging using contrast-enhanced CT angiography and MR angiography is becoming increasingly useful, particularly in neonates where the risk of catheter angiography is greatest. However, digital subtraction cerebral angiography is best for precise evaluation of vascular architecture in VOGMs [189].

Fetal ultrasound and MRI are useful for the antenatal diagnosis of aneurysmal malformations of the Vein of Galen, and allow for early management decisions to be made [190-192].

4.5 Treatment and prognosis

Many patients are not offered invasive treatment for their VOGM, usually due to poor cardiac or neurological condition at the time of diagnosis. Without treatment, VOGM is associated with a fatal outcome in >90% [193], usually from cardiac failure or neurological complications such as hydrocephalus.

Treatments strategies have evolved dramatically over the past decades, with series published before the year 2000 reporting a 15% mortality rate with endovascular management, and an 85% mortality rate with microsurgical management [193]. For this reason, surgery is rarely recommended as a first-line management option for VOGM. Although ventricular shunting may be required for the management of hydrocephalus in older children and adults, this may be avoided with early endovascular occlusion of the arteriovenous shunt in neonates and infants [194]. The published experience on stereotactic radiosurgery for VOGM is extremely limited [195].

Endovascular approaches to treatment are usually performed with the goal of obtaining complete exclusion of the malformation through a combination of transarterial and transvenous routes (with transarterial being the preferred route, and transvenous access only required in 2%) [194]. Multiple treatment sessions are usually required (average 2.4 sessions per child), and total or near-total occlusion was obtained in 55% of patients in this series.

Although published series in the past 10 years have not reported a change in the mortality rate significantly [193], the extensive experience reported from the Hospital de Bicetre, France, describes good clinical outcomes in 74% of patients and a mortality rate of 11% [194].

Outcome from endovascular treatment is highly dependent on the age of the patient at the time of presentation. Mortality rates as high as 50% have been recorded in neonates, with death rates around 7% in infants (<2 yrs) and 0-3% in children and adults undergoing treatment [193, 194].

4.6 Screening of relatives

There is no evidence to suggest that antenatal diagnosis of VOGM is associated with improved treatment outcomes, although it may assist with early referral to a center with experience in management of the complex cardiac and neurological issues facing these patients [192]. In spite of this, there is currently no evidence to support the use of diagnostic imaging to screen for the presence of VOMG in asymptomatic patients.

5. Capillary telangiectasia

5.1 Theories of pathogenesis

Capillary telangiectasias consist of multiple abnormally dilated capillary vessels, with normal intervening brain parenchyma. They are relatively common, rarely symptomatic, and are most commonly found in the region of the pons [196, 197]. They are traditionally considered to be congenital malformations, arising as a result of aberrant angiogenesis or failure of capillary involution during development [198]. This belief is based on the assumption that brain capillary telangiectasias are the same as cutaneous capillary malformations (or 'port wine stains') [29], although little evidence exists to support this theory of pathogenesis. Capillary telangiectasias have been reported to co-exist with developmental venous anomalies and cerebral cavernous malformations [198, 199], as well as developing after resection of a cavernous malformation [213]. This last case in particular indicates that *de novo* capillary telangiectasias may develop in adults, and suggests that these lesions may represent a spectrum of the same disease process.

5.2 Genetics

Although several genetic loci have been implicated in the development of cutaneous capillary malformations (including mutations of the RASA1 gene, located on chromosome 5q13-22, and implicated in Parkes-Weber Syndrome, a condition associated with cutaneous capillary malformations and brain AVMs) [187], very little is known about the role of genetic abnormalities in capillary telangiectasias of the brain.

5.3 Clinical features

It is very rare for capillary telangiectasias to present clinically; they are often found as an incidental finding at autopsy or during MR imaging for other unrelated conditions [197, 200]. Occasionally, they can present with hemorrhage or mass effect on surrounding structures, resulting in seizures, cranial nerve dysfunction, confusion, dizziness, visual disturbance, vertigo, tinnitus, or motor deficits [200, 201]. They have been implicated as a potential cause of non-aneurysmal perimesencephalic subarachnoid hemorrhage [202].

5.4 Diagnosis, including early detection

Brain capillary telangiectasias are not seen on CT, and are difficult to detect on MRI with standard T1- and T2- weighted imaging. However, they display mild homogenous enhancement with contrast material, and are often markedly hypo-intense on Gradient Echo sequences [200, 203]. They are not demonstrable on digital subtraction cerebral angiography.

5.5 Treatment

It is extremely rare for small brain capillary telangiectasias (<1 cm in maximum dimension) to present with symptoms, and the majority of cases do not require active treatment. Larger lesions may be symptomatic, and require surgical resection [200].

5.6 Prognosis

Capillary telangiectasias are benign lesions that usually do not cause neurological symptoms. In a large series of over 100 patients with brain capillary telangiectasias, only 2 patients were symptomatic, and 1 patient required surgical resection [200]. Other smaller series have reported on lesions where symptoms have improved with medical management of seizures, or have resolved spontaneously [201]. Rarely have reports described progressive neurological symptoms or death from unruptured capillary telangiectasias [204, 205]. Although hemorrhage from a capillary telangiectasia has been reported [202], the risk of hemorrhagic complications from these lesions is not known.

5.7 Screening of relatives

There is no evidence to support the use of diagnostic imaging to screen for the presence of capillary telangiectasias in asymptomatic patients.

6. Cavernous malformation

6.1 Theories of pathogenesis

Cavernous malformations (cavernomas, cavernous hemangioma) consist of abnormal, thin-walled sinusoidal vascular channels. There is not generally any brain parenchyma between the vessels and there is lack of basement membrane, smooth muscle, elastin, and adventitia [228,229]. Most cases have either imaging or pathological evidence of prior hemorrhage and organizing thrombus; calcification is also frequently seen.

As with other vascular malformations described in this chapter, there was an initial assumption of a congenital origin, which has recently been brought in to question. New malformations have been documented in familial and non-familial cases and in regions of brain treated with radiotherapy for other conditions [228]. Genetic abnormalities have been identified in patients with familial cavernous malformations. The genes identified code for proteins that are important for vascular development.

Another proposed mechanism of cavernous malformation development is venous hypertension, particularly in cases associated with developmental venous anomalies [232]. The proposal is that chronically raised venous pressure influences the development of cavernous malformations or may at least predispose to their recurrence after surgical removal.

6.2 Genetics

Cavernous malformations occur in all races and there is no sex predilection. The prevalence is approximately 0.5% [228], although the rate is higher in the Hispanic population. In some familial forms there is almost 100% penetrance [228]. Almost all Hispanic patients and 40% of Caucasian patients with familial cavernous malformations have a constitutional defect in the KRIT1 gene, also known as CCM1 [230]. KRIT1 codes for a protein that plays an important role in blood vessel development and may play a role in blood-brain-barrier formation. Over 100 mutations of the KRIT1 gene have been identified that are associated with the development of cavernous malformations.

Defects in other genes, (CCM2 and CCM3), are also associated with cavernous malformation development. CCM2 and CCM3 code for proteins that are thought to be important in the signaling between neurons and developing vascular cells in the central nervous system. Many different mutations of these genes have been identified in cavernous malformation patients, accounting for approximately one third of familial cases [231].

6.3 Clinical features

Cavernous malformations account for up to 10% of central nervous system vascular malformations and the mean age at presentation is approximately 40 [228]. In familial cases there are often multiple lesions, whereas sporadic cases usually have only one lesion.

Presentation is with headache or neurological deficit from hemorrhage, or with seizures. In contrast to AVMs, hemorrhages from cavernous malformations are generally not life-threatening. Neurological deficits occur when the lesions are in eloquent regions of the brain such as the brain stem or primary motor cortex. The annual risk of hemorrhage has been estimated at 4%, with higher risks accompanying familial cases, after an initial clinical hemorrhage, or for lesions located in the brain stem [228]. There may be a higher risk during pregnancy.

6.4 Diagnosis, including early detection

Catheter angiography will often not reveal cavernous malformations. Subtle hyperdensity may be seen on non-contrast CT, although even a contrast scan will not detect many lesions. The hemosiderin deposition resulting from prior hemorrhages makes MRI an exquisitely sensitive diagnostic technique. In addition to making the diagnosis, MRI is important for determining the location of the lesion and its relationship to pial or ependymal surfaces, which are important factors in surgical decision-making.

6.5 Treatment

Surgical excision is the only effective treatment for cavernous malformations; there is no role for endovascular therapy and there is little evidence supporting the efficacy of radiosurgery. The indications for surgery are to prevent hemorrhage and to improve control of seizures. Excision of lesions in asymptomatic patients is usually not justified. Surgery is reasonable for lesions in the brain stem that have bled at least once, and where the lesion comes to either a pial or ependymal surface. If seizure control is the main concern, it may be preferable to proceed with surgery within the first year after presentation, as there is some evidence that this improves seizure outcomes [228].

6.6 Prognosis

Left untreated, cavernous malformations remain at risk of hemorrhage. Neurological deficits are particularly common after hemorrhage in the brain stem and the effects are cumulative with each hemorrhage. Surgical excision of cavernous malformations relieves mass effect on surrounding brain and may be effective in controlling seizures, especially if surrounding hemosiderin-stained tissue is removed. Unfortunately, removal of lesions in the brain stem does not necessarily eliminate the risk of hemorrhage: there is a growing awareness of a moderately high rate of recurrence in this region and the spinal cord [233]. Whether recurrence is related to further growth of residual malformation or development of a new lesion remains to be determined.

6.7 Screening of relatives

Although familial forms of the condition are well recognized, there is not a clear indication for screening relatives of affected patients. Since there is not usually an indication for treatment of asymptomatic patients with cavernous malformations of the brain, we do not generally recommend screening. For relatives in familial cases who request screening, it is reasonable to obtain an MR scan.

7. Developmental venous anomalies

7.1 Theories of pathogenesis

Developmental venous anomalies (also known as developmental venous malformations and venous angiomas) are composed of a radially-arranged cluster of venous radicles converging into a larger, mature venous channel [206, 207]. The venous structures are angiographically mature, and express normal structural proteins in their walls [208].

There are several broad theories of pathogenesis for DVAs, and all assume that they form *in utero*. The first theory is that DVAs represent anatomical variants formed by the opening of transhemispheric anastomotic pathways between the superficial venous system and the deep venous system of the brain in response to hemodynamic demand [209]. In this model, the DVA is a normal structure, performing a normal physiological function.

Other theories propose that DVAs form in response to thrombosis or occlusion of normal parenchymal veins, or as a result of abnormal fetal angiogenesis [210, 211]. These theories consider the DVA to be a response to an antenatal pathological event rather than a normal anatomical variant [212].

7.2 Genetics

Developmental venous anomalies are associated with other cerebral vascular malformations, in particular cerebral cavernous malformations, in up to 40% of cases [206]. Isolated case reports have described the temporal development of a cerebral cavernous malformation in the region of a DVA; prompting the suggestion that regional venous hypertension may serve as a common pathogenetic mechanism [213, 214]. Familial cavernous malformations are unlikely to be associated with the presence of a DVA, whereas a DVA is likely to co-exist with a sporadic CCM in almost half of cases [215], countering the argument that a simple genetic defect is responsible for the co-existence of these two vascular malformations.

Intracranial DVAs are also associated with peripheral vascular abnormalities, and are present in 20% of patients with cutaneous venous malformations [207]. In particular, DVAs have been reported in patients with blue rubber bleb nevus syndrome and sinus pericranii, prompting the suggestion that sinus pericranii should be considered the extracranial manifestation of a common spectrum of venous malformations [216, 217].

The vast majority (about 95%) of cutaneous venous malformations are sporadic, but a small proportion of cutaneomucosal venous malformations are inherited in an autosomal dominant pattern. The genetic defect responsible for this form of venous malformations is a mutation in the TEK gene (encoding for the angiopoieten receptor, TIE2; located on chromosome 9p21) [218, 219]. Despite the potential for a link between these malformations and DVAs, there is no evidence to support the hypothesis that this gene defect is responsible for the development of intracranial DVAs.

Intracranial DVAs have also been reported in associated with the spectrum of vascular anomalies occurring in patients with mutations of the PTEN gene [220].

7.3 Clinical features

Developmental venous anomalies are the most common cerebral vascular malformation, with a prevalence in imaging series of 0.5-0.7%, and in autopsy series of 2.6% [207]. The vast majority are asymptomatic, and are often found as an incidental finding during imaging for other unrelated conditions.

The most common reason for neuroimaging in patients with a DVA is headache; however, an exact causal relationship is often difficult to prove, as symptoms may resolve over time without treatment of the vascular anomaly. Similarly, in patients presenting with seizure or neurological deficit, there is often no direct correlation between the anatomical location of the DVA and the neurological symptoms [207].

The risk of hemorrhage from a DVA is low, with retrospective series reporting an annual hemorrhage rate of 0.6%, and prospective series reporting an annual hemorrhage rate of 0.7% (with a symptomatic hemorrhage rate of 0.3%) [221]. Cerebral edema, venous infarction, and hemorrhage may occur following stenosis or thrombosis of the draining vein of the DVA [212, 222].

7.4 Diagnosis, including early detection

Developmental venous anomalies are rarely visible on non-contrast CT imaging, unless associated with a cavernous malformation. Following the administration of intravenous contrast, the DVA is visualized as a collection of venous tributaries or 'caput medusa' draining via an enlarged draining vein [214]. CT perfusion studies may be useful in determining the hemodynamic alterations present as a result of the altered regional venous drainage [223].

Similarly, DVAs may be seen on T1- and T2-weighted MR imaging, but are best visualized on gadolinium-enhanced T1-weighted imaging. Gradient echo sequences may show a ring of hypointensity if previous hemorrhage or an associated cavernous malformation is present. MR imaging is also valuable for the detection of parenchymal abnormalities often associated with DVAs [214].

Conventional digital subtraction angiography shows normal arterial and capillary phase, with typical venous phase demonstrating the 'caput meduase' of dilated medullary veins converging upon an enlarged subcortical or subependymal draining vein [207, 224]

7.5 Treatment

Traditionally, neurosurgeons have understood that DVAs represent a variant of normal venous drainage, and as such should never be a target for treatment [209]. However, others have challenged this belief, suggesting that removal of CCM without removal of the underlying DVA results in recurrence of the CCM in up to one third of patients. Particularly in this group of patients, cautious coagulation and dissection of the large transcerebral DVA may be considered [225].

We advocate a conservative approach, and recommend that surgical treatment never be offered to patients with asymptomatic DVAs. In the setting where hemorrhage has occurred, then evacuation of the hematoma may be considered, but surgical disruption of the DVA should be avoided. Associated cavernous malformations should be completely excised, with preservation of the anomalous venous drainage wherever possible. We do not believe that sufficient evidence exists to support the routine removal of DVAs to prevent the development of recurrent cavernous malformation.

7.6 Prognosis

Most of the evidence relating to DVAs suggests that they are a variant of normal venous drainage; they are a normal structure, performing a normal physiological function. Once considered a rarity, with a high propensity for hemorrhage, they are in fact the most frequently encountered vascular malformation, occurring in up to 3% of the population [226]. Developmental venous anomalies themselves have a very low risk of hemorrhage, with prospective series reporting a symptomatic hemorrhage rate as low as 0.3% [221]. They are, however, associated with the development of other vascular malformations (in particular cavernous malformation), which increase the risk of symptomatic hemorrhage to as high as 6% per year [227].

7.7 Screening of relatives

There is currently no evidence to support the use of diagnostic imaging to screen for the presence of DVAs in asymptomatic patients. Although of little clinical benefit, there may be research interest in screening relatives of patients with blue rubber-bleb nevus syndrome for intracranial venous anomalies, in order to improve our understanding of the genetic and molecular influences responsible for the development of vascular malformations in these patients.

8. References

[1] Streeter, G.L., *The development of the venous sinsues of the dural mater in the human embryo.* Am J Anat, 1915. 18(2): p. 145-178.

[2] Streeter, G.L., *The developmental alterations in the vascular system of the brain of the human embryo.* Contrib Embryol, 1918. 8: p. 5-38.

[3] Padget, D.H., *The development of the cranial arteries in the human embryo.* Contrib Embryol, 1948. 32: p. 205-263.

[4] Padget, D.H., *The cranial venous system in man in reference to development, adult configuration, and relation to the arteries.* Am J Anat, 1956. 98(3): p. 307-55.

[5] Padget, D.H., *The development of the cranial venous system in man, from the viewpoint of comparative anatomy.* Contrib Embryol, 1957. 247: p. 81-139.

[6] Davidson, A.S. and M.K. Morgan, *The embryologic basis for the anatomy of the cerebral vasculature related to arteriovenous malformations.* J Clin Neurosci, 2011. 18(4): p. 464-9.

[7] Velut, S., *[Embryology of the cerebral veins].* Neurochirurgie, 1987. 33(4): p. 258-63.

[8] Mullan, S., et al., *Embryological basis of some aspects of cerebral vascular fistulas and malformations.* J Neurosurg, 1996. 85(1): p. 1-8.

[9] Truwit, C.L., *Embryology of the cerebral vasculature.* Neuroimaging Clin N Am, 1994. 4(4): p. 663-89.

[10] Raybaud, C.A., et al., *[Aneurysms of the vein of Galen. Angiographic study and morphogenetic considerations].* Neurochirurgie, 1987. 33(4): p. 302-14.

[11] Yasargil, M.G., *Microneurosurgery Vol IIIA: AVM of the brain, history, embryology, pathological considerations, hemodynamics, diagnostic studies, microsurgical anatomy.* Microneurosurgery, ed. M.G. Yasargil. Vol. IIIA. 1987, New York: Thieme Medical Publishers. 408.

[12] Warkany, J. and R.J. Lemire, *Arteriovenous malformations of the brain: a teratologic challenge.* Teratology, 1984. 29(3): p. 333-53.

[13] Kim, H., et al., *Comparison of 2 approaches for determining the natural history risk of brain arteriovenous malformation rupture.* Am J Epidemiol, 2010. 171(12): p. 1317-22.

[14] Kim, H., et al., *Brain arteriovenous malformation biology relevant to hemorrhage and implication for therapeutic development.* Stroke, 2009. 40(3 Suppl): p. S95-7.

[15] Kim, H., et al., *Genetic considerations relevant to intracranial hemorrhage and brain arteriovenous malformations.* Acta Neurochir Suppl, 2008. 105: p. 199-206.

[16] Jeffree, R.L. and M.A. Stoodley, *Postnatal development of arteriovenous malformations.* Pediatr Neurosurg, 2009. 45(4): p. 296-304.

[17] Stapf, C. and J.P. Mohr, *New concepts in adult brain arteriovenous malformations.* Curr Opin Neurol, 2000. 13(1): p. 63-7.

[18] van Beijnum, J., et al., *Familial occurrence of brain arteriovenous malformations: a systematic review.* J Neurol Neurosurg Psychiatry, 2007. 78(11): p. 1213-7.
[19] Inoue, S., et al., *Combination of linkage and association studies for brain arteriovenous malformation.* Stroke, 2007. 38(4): p. 1368-70.
[20] Henn, J.S., S. Coons, and J.M. Zabramski, *Pathology and classification of central nervous system vascular malformations,* in *Vascular malformations of the central nervous system,* J.J. Jafar, I.A. Awad, and R.H. Rosenwasser, Editors. 1999, Lippincott Williams & Wilkins: Philadelphia. p. 71-94.
[21] Letteboer, T.G., et al., *Genotype-phenotype relationship in hereditary haemorrhagic telangiectasia.* J Med Genet, 2006. 43(4): p. 371-7.
[22] Govani, F.S. and C.L. Shovlin, *Hereditary haemorrhagic telangiectasia: a clinical and scientific review.* Eur J Hum Genet, 2009. 17(7): p. 860-71.
[23] Matsubara, S., et al., *Angiographic and clinical characteristics of patients with cerebral arteriovenous malformations associated with hereditary hemorrhagic telangiectasia.* AJNR Am J Neuroradiol, 2000. 21(6): p. 1016-20.
[24] Willinsky, R.A., et al., *Multiple cerebral arteriovenous malformations (AVMs). Review of our experience from 203 patients with cerebral vascular lesions.* Neuroradiology, 1990. 32(3): p. 207-10.
[25] Berman, M.F., et al., *The epidemiology of brain arteriovenous malformations.* Neurosurgery, 2000. 47(2): p. 389-96; discussion 397.
[26] Toporsian, M. and M. Letarte, *Hereditary hemorrhagic telangiectasia: A model to probe the biology of the vascular endothelium,* in *Endothelial Biomedicine,* W.C. Aird, Editor 2007, Cambridge University Press: New York. p. 1113-1123.
[27] Putman, C.M., et al., *Exceptional multiplicity of cerebral arteriovenous malformations associated with hereditary hemorrhagic telangiectasia (Osler-Weber-Rendu syndrome).* AJNR Am J Neuroradiol, 1996. 17(9): p. 1733-42.
[28] Du, R., et al., *Growth and regression of arteriovenous malformations in a patient with hereditary hemorrhagic telangiectasia. Case report.* J Neurosurg, 2007. 106(3): p. 470-7.
[29] Garzon, M.C., et al., *Vascular malformations. Part II: associated syndromes.* J Am Acad Dermatol, 2007. 56(4): p. 541-64.
[30] Dayani, P.N. and A.A. Sadun, *A case report of Wyburn-Mason syndrome and review of the literature.* Neuroradiology, 2007. 49(5): p. 445-56.
[31] Comi, A.M., *Update on Sturge-Weber syndrome: diagnosis, treatment, quantitative measures, and controversies.* Lymphat Res Biol, 2007. 5(4): p. 257-64.
[32] Hashimoto, T., et al., *Gene microarray analysis of human brain arteriovenous malformations.* Neurosurgery, 2004. 54(2): p. 410-23; discussion 423-5.
[33] Hashimoto, T., et al., *Abnormal balance in the angiopoietin-tie2 system in human brain arteriovenous malformations.* Circ Res, 2001. 89(2): p. 111-3.
[34] Shenkar, R., et al., *Differential gene expression in human cerebrovascular malformations.* Neurosurgery, 2003. 52(2): p. 465-77; discussion 477-8.
[35] Sasahara, A., et al., *Increased expression of ephrin A1 in brain arteriovenous malformation: DNA microarray analysis.* Neurosurg Rev, 2007. 30(4): p. 299-305; discussion 305.
[36] Kim, H., et al., *Common variants in interleukin-1-Beta gene are associated with intracranial hemorrhage and susceptibility to brain arteriovenous malformation.* Cerebrovasc Dis, 2009. 27(2): p. 176-82.

[37] Pawlikowska, L., et al., *Polymorphisms in genes involved in inflammatory and angiogenic pathways and the risk of hemorrhagic presentation of brain arteriovenous malformations.* Stroke, 2004. 35(10): p. 2294-300.

[38] Pawlikowska, L., et al., *Apolipoprotein E epsilon 2 is associated with new hemorrhage risk in brain arteriovenous malformations.* Neurosurgery, 2006. 58(5): p. 838-43; discussion 838-43.

[39] Achrol, A.S., et al., *Tumor necrosis factor-alpha-238G>A promoter polymorphism is associated with increased risk of new hemorrhage in the natural course of patients with brain arteriovenous malformations.* Stroke, 2006. 37(1): p. 231-4.

[40] da Costa, L., et al., *The natural history and predictive features of hemorrhage from brain arteriovenous malformations.* Stroke, 2009. 40(1): p. 100-5.

[41] Graf, C.J., G.E. Perret, and J.C. Torner, *Bleeding from cerebral arteriovenous malformations as part of their natural history.* J Neurosurg, 1983. 58(3): p. 331-7.

[42] Brown, R.D., Jr., et al., *The natural history of unruptured intracranial arteriovenous malformations.* J Neurosurg, 1988. 68(3): p. 352-7.

[43] Ondra, S.L., et al., *The natural history of symptomatic arteriovenous malformations of the brain: a 24-year follow-up assessment.* J Neurosurg, 1990. 73(3): p. 387-91.

[44] Halim, A.X., et al., *Longitudinal risk of intracranial hemorrhage in patients with arteriovenous malformation of the brain within a defined population.* Stroke, 2004. 35(7): p. 1697-702.

[45] Stapf, C., et al., *Predictors of hemorrhage in patients with untreated brain arteriovenous malformation.* Neurology, 2006. 66(9): p. 1350-5.

[46] Hernesniemi, J.A., et al., *Natural history of brain arteriovenous malformations: a long-term follow-up study of risk of hemorrhage in 238 patients.* Neurosurgery, 2008. 63(5): p. 823-9; discussion 829-31.

[47] Al-Shahi, R., et al., *Prospective, population-based detection of intracranial vascular malformations in adults: the Scottish Intracranial Vascular Malformation Study (SIVMS).* Stroke, 2003. 34(5): p. 1163-9.

[48] Hillman, J., *Population-based analysis of arteriovenous malformation treatment.* J Neurosurg, 2001. 95(4): p. 633-7.

[49] ApSimon, H.T., et al., *A population-based study of brain arteriovenous malformation: long-term treatment outcomes.* Stroke, 2002. 33(12): p. 2794-800.

[50] Stapf, C., et al., *The New York Islands AVM Study: design, study progress, and initial results.* Stroke, 2003. 34(5): p. e29-33.

[51] Gabriel, R.A., et al., *Ten-year detection rate of brain arteriovenous malformations in a large, multiethnic, defined population.* Stroke, 2010. 41(1): p. 21-6.

[52] Choi, J.H., et al., *Clinical and morphological determinants of focal neurological deficits in patients with unruptured brain arteriovenous malformation.* J Neurol Sci, 2009. 287(1-2): p. 126-30.

[53] Haas, D.C., *Arteriovenous malformations and migraine: case reports and an analysis of the relationship.* Headache, 1991. 31(8): p. 509-13.

[54] Monteiro, J.M., et al., *Migraine and intracranial vascular malformations.* Headache, 1993. 33(10): p. 563-5.

[55] Bruyn, G.W., *Intracranial arteriovenous malformation and migraine.* Cephalalgia, 1984. 4(3): p. 191-207.

[56] Morris, Z., et al., *Incidental findings on brain magnetic resonance imaging: systematic review and meta-analysis.* BMJ, 2009. 339: p. b3016.

[57] Al-Shahi, R. and C. Warlow, *A systematic review of the frequency and prognosis of arteriovenous malformations of the brain in adults.* Brain, 2001. 124(Pt 10): p. 1900-26.
[58] Ducreux, D., et al., *[Diffusion, perfusion and activation functional MRI studies of brain arteriovenous malformations].* J Neuroradiol, 2004. 31(1): p. 25-34.
[59] Yamada, K., et al., *Tractography for arteriovenous malformations near the sensorimotor cortices.* AJNR Am J Neuroradiol, 2005. 26(3): p. 598-602.
[60] Strozyk, D., R.G. Nogueira, and S.D. Lavine, *Endovascular treatment of intracranial arteriovenous malformation.* Neurosurg Clin N Am, 2009. 20(4): p. 399-418.
[61] Smith, C.M., *Origin and uses of primum non nocere--above all, do no harm!* J Clin Pharmacol, 2005. 45(4): p. 371-7.
[62] Mast, H., et al., *Risk of spontaneous haemorrhage after diagnosis of cerebral arteriovenous malformation.* Lancet, 1997. 350(9084): p. 1065-8.
[63] Yamada, S., et al., *Risk factors for subsequent hemorrhage in patients with cerebral arteriovenous malformations.* J Neurosurg, 2007. 107(5): p. 965-72.
[64] Perret, G. and H. Nishioka, *Report on the cooperative study of intracranial aneurysms and subarachnoid hemorrhage. Section VI. Arteriovenous malformations. An analysis of 545 cases of cranio-cerebral arteriovenous malformations and fistulae reported to the cooperative study.* J Neurosurg, 1966. 25(4): p. 467-90.
[65] Choi, J.H., et al., *Clinical outcome after first and recurrent hemorrhage in patients with untreated brain arteriovenous malformation.* Stroke, 2006. 37(5): p. 1243-7.
[66] Rankin, J., *Cerebral vascular accidents in patients over the age of 60. Prognosis.* Scottish Medical Journal, 1957. 2(5): p. 200-15.
[67] Laakso, A., et al., *Long-term excess mortality in 623 patients with brain arteriovenous malformations.* Neurosurgery, 2008. 63(2): p. 244-53; discussion 253-5.
[68] Morgan, M.K., et al., *Surgical risks associated with the management of Grade I and II brain arteriovenous malformations.* Neurosurgery, 2004. 54(4): p. 832-7.
[69] Hashimoto, N., et al., *Surgery of cerebral arteriovenous malformations.* Neurosurgery, 2007. 61(1 Suppl): p. 375-87; discussion 387-9.
[70] Zhao, J., et al., *Clinical characteristics and surgical results of patients with cerebral arteriovenous malformations.* Surg Neurol, 2005. 63(2): p. 156-61; discussion 161.
[71] Hernesniemi, J., et al., *Present state of microneurosurgery of cerebral arteriovenous malformations.* Acta Neurochir Suppl, 2010. 107: p. 71-6.
[72] Morgan, M.K., *Classification and decision making in treatment and perioperative management, including surgical and radiosurgical decision making,* in *Youmans Neurological Surgery,* H.R. Winn, Editor 2004, Elsevier Inc.: Philadelphia. p. 2185-2204.
[73] Morgan, M.K., et al., *Surgery for cerebral arteriovenous malformation: risks related to lenticulostriate arterial supply.* Journal of Neurosurgery, 1997. 86(5): p. 801-5.
[74] Lawton, M.T., *Spetzler-Martin Grade III arteriovenous malformations: surgical results and a modification of the grading scale.* Neurosurgery, 2003. 52(4): p. 740-8; discussion 748-9.
[75] Han, P.P., F.A. Ponce, and R.F. Spetzler, *Intention-to-treat analysis of Spetzler-Martin grades IV and V arteriovenous malformations: natural history and treatment paradigm.* J Neurosurg, 2003. 98(1): p. 3-7.
[76] Chang, S.D., et al., *Multimodality treatment of giant intracranial arteriovenous malformations.* Neurosurgery, 2003. 53(1): p. 1-11; discussion 11-3.
[77] Ferch, R.D. and M.K. Morgan, *High-grade arteriovenous malformations and their management.* J Clin Neurosci, 2002. 9(1): p. 37-40.

[78] Morgan, M.K., et al., *Delayed hemorrhage following resection of an arteriovenous malformation in the brain.* J Neurosurg, 2003. 99(6): p. 967-71.

[79] Lawton, M.T., et al., *A supplementary grading scale for selecting patients with brain arteriovenous malformations for surgery.* Neurosurgery, 2010. 66(4): p. 702-13; discussion 713.

[80] Zhao, J., et al., *Surgical treatment of giant intracranial arteriovenous malformations.* Neurosurgery, 2010. 67(5): p. 1359-70; discussion 1370.

[81] Joaquim, A.F. and E. de Oliveira, *Management of supratentorial arteriovenous malformations.* Clin Neurosurg, 2009. 56: p. 40-4.

[82] Davidson, A.S. and M.K. Morgan, *How safe is arteriovenous malformation surgery? A prospective, observational study of surgery as first-line treatment for brain arteriovenous malformations.* Neurosurgery, 2010. 66(3): p. 498-504; discussion 504-5.

[83] Friedman, W.A., *Linear accelerator radiosurgery*, in *Principles and practice of stereotactic radiosurgery*, L.S. Chin and W.F. Regine, Editors. 2008, Springer: New York. p. 129-140.

[84] Han, J.H., et al., *Clinical and neuroimaging outcome of cerebral arteriovenous malformations after Gamma Knife surgery: analysis of the radiation injury rate depending on the arteriovenous malformation volume.* J Neurosurg, 2008. 109(2): p. 191-8.

[85] Starke, R.M., et al., *A comprehensive review of radiosurgery for cerebral arteriovenous malformations: outcomes, predictive factors, and grading scales.* Stereotact Funct Neurosurg, 2008. 86(3): p. 191-9.

[86] Colombo, F., et al., *Early results of CyberKnife radiosurgery for arteriovenous malformations.* J Neurosurg, 2009. 111(4): p. 807-19.

[87] Raffa, S.J., et al., *Validation of the radiosurgery-based arteriovenous malformation score in a large linear accelerator radiosurgery experience.* J Neurosurg, 2009. 111(4): p. 832-9.

[88] Zabel, A., et al., *Treatment outcome after linac-based radiosurgery in cerebral arteriovenous malformations: retrospective analysis of factors affecting obliteration.* Radiother Oncol, 2005. 77(1): p. 105-10.

[89] Maruyama, K., et al., *The risk of hemorrhage after radiosurgery for cerebral arteriovenous malformations.* N Engl J Med, 2005. 352(2): p. 146-53.

[90] Andrade-Souza, Y.M., et al., *Testing the radiosurgery-based arteriovenous malformation score and the modified Spetzler-Martin grading system to predict radiosurgical outcome.* J Neurosurg, 2005. 103(4): p. 642-8.

[91] Wegner, R.E., et al., *A Modified Radiosurgery-Based Arteriovenous Malformation Grading Scale and Its Correlation with Outcomes.* Int J Radiat Oncol Biol Phys, 2011. 79(4): p. 1147-1150.

[92] Panagiotopoulos, V., et al., *Embolization of intracranial arteriovenous malformations with ethylene-vinyl alcohol copolymer (Onyx).* AJNR Am J Neuroradiol, 2009. 30(1): p. 99-106.

[93] Xu, F., et al., *Onyx embolization for the treatment of brain arteriovenous malformations.* Acta Neurochir (Wien), 2010.

[94] Katsaridis, V., C. Papagiannaki, and E. Aimar, *Curative embolization of cerebral arteriovenous malformations (AVMs) with Onyx in 101 patients.* Neuroradiology, 2008. 50(7): p. 589-97.

[95] Weber, W., et al., *Preoperative embolization of intracranial arteriovenous malformations with Onyx.* Neurosurgery, 2007. 61(2): p. 244-52; discussion 252-4.

[96] van Rooij, W.J., M. Sluzewski, and G.N. Beute, *Brain AVM embolization with Onyx.* AJNR Am J Neuroradiol, 2007. 28(1): p. 172-7; discussion 178.
[97] Xu, F., et al., *Onyx embolization for the treatment of brain arteriovenous malformations.* Acta Neurochir (Wien), 2011. 153(4): p. 869-78.
[98] Saatci, I., et al., *Endovascular treatment of brain arteriovenous malformations with prolonged intranidal Onyx injection technique: long-term results in 350 consecutive patients with completed endovascular treatment course.* J Neurosurg, 2011. 115(1): p. 78-88.
[99] Easey, A.J., et al., *Should asymptomatic patients with hereditary haemorrhagic telangiectasia (HHT) be screened for cerebral vascular malformations? Data from 22,061 years of HHT patient life.* J Neurol Neurosurg Psychiatry, 2003. 74(6): p. 743-8.
[100] Gordon, I.J., et al., *Giant dural supratentorial arteriovenous malformation.* AJR. American Journal of Roentgenology, 1977. 129(4): p. 734-6.
[101] Grisoli, F., et al., *Surgical treatment of tentorial arteriovenous malformations draining into the subarachnoid space. Report of four cases.* Journal of Neurosurgery, 1984. 60(5): p. 1059-66.
[102] Newton, T.H. and S. Cronqvist, *Involvement of dural arteries in intracranial arteriovenous malformations.* Radiology, 1969. 93(5): p. 1071-8.
[103] Vidyasagar, C., *Persistent embryonic veins in the arteriovenous malformations of the dura.* Acta Neurochirurgica, 1979. 48(3-4): p. 199-216.
[104] Obrador, S., M. Soto, and J. Silvela, *Clinical syndromes of arteriovenous malformations of the transverse-sigmoid sinus.* Journal of Neurology, Neurosurgery & Psychiatry, 1975. 38(5): p. 436-51.
[105] Lasjaunias, P., et al., *Anatomoclinical aspects of dural arteriovenous shunts in children.* Interventional Neuroradiology, 1996. 2: p. 179-191.
[106] Cognard, C., et al., *Cerebral dural arteriovenous fistulas: clinical and angiographic correlation with a revised classification of venous drainage.* Radiology, 1995. 194(3): p. 671-80.
[107] Davies, M.A., et al., *The validity of classification for the clinical presentation of intracranial dural arteriovenous fistulas.* Journal of Neurosurgery, 1996. 85(5): p. 830-7.
[108] Kim, M.S., et al., *Clinical characteristics of dural arteriovenous fistula.* Journal of Clinical Neuroscience, 2002. 9(2): p. 147-55.
[109] Urtasun, F., et al., *Cerebral dural arteriovenous fistulas: percutaneous transvenous embolization.* Radiology, 1996. 199(1): p. 209-17.
[110] Lucas, C.P., et al., *Treatment for intracranial dural arteriovenous malformations: a meta-analysis from the English language literature.* Neurosurgery, 1997. 40(6): p. 1119-30; discussion 1130-2.
[111] Houser, O.W., et al., *Arteriovenous malformation affecting the transverse dural venous sinus--an acquired lesion.* Mayo Clinic Proceedings, 1979. 54(10): p. 651-61.
[112] Brainin, M. and P. Samec, *Venous hemodynamics of arteriovenous meningeal fistulas in the posterior cranial fossa.* Neuroradiology, 1983. 25(3): p. 161-9.
[113] Piton, J., et al., *Fistulae of the lateral sinus.* Journal of Neuroradiology. Journal de Neuroradiologie, 1984. 11(3): p. 143-59.
[114] Mizutani, T., H. Tanaka, and T. Aruga, *Multiple arteriovenous malformations located in the cerebellum, posterior fossa, spinal cord, dura, and scalp with associated port-wine stain and supratentorial venous anomaly.* Neurosurgery, 1992. 31(1): p. 137-40; discussion 140-1.

[115] Carvalho, S., et al., *Blue rubber-bleb nevus syndrome: report of a familial case with a dural arteriovenous fistula.* Ajnr: American Journal of Neuroradiology, 2003. 24(9): p. 1916-8.

[116] Cataltepe, O., et al., *An unusual dural arteriovenous fistula in an infant.* Neuroradiology, 1993. 35(5): p. 394-7.

[117] Debrun, G.M., et al., *Indications for treatment and classification of 132 carotid-cavernous fistulas.* Neurosurgery, 1988. 22(2): p. 285-9.

[118] Halbach, V.V., et al., *Treatment of carotid-cavernous fistulas associated with Ehlers-Danlos syndrome.* Neurosurgery, 1990. 26(6): p. 1021-7.

[119] Schievink, W.I., et al., *Spontaneous carotid-cavernous fistulae in Ehlers-Danlos syndrome Type IV. Case report.* Journal of Neurosurgery, 1991. 74(6): p. 991-8.

[120] Mullan, S., *Treatment of carotid-cavernous fistulas by cavernous sinus occlusion.* Journal of Neurosurgery, 1979. 50(2): p. 131-44.

[121] Hieshima, G.B., et al., *Spontaneous arteriovenous fistulas of cerebral vessels in association with fibromuscular dysplasia.* Neurosurgery, 1986. 18(4): p. 454-8.

[122] Hieshima, G.B., et al., *Calvarial, orbital and dural vascular anomalies in hereditary hemorrhagic telangiectasia.* Surgical Neurology, 1977. 8(4): p. 263-7.

[123] Maher, C.O., et al., *Cerebrovascular manifestations in 321 cases of hereditary hemorrhagic telangiectasia.[see comment].* Stroke, 2001. 32(4): p. 877-82.

[124] Ng, P., et al., *Endovascular strategies for carotid cavernous and intracerebral dural arteriovenous fistulas.* Neurosurgery Focus, 2003. 15(4): p. 1-6.

[125] Rumboldt, Z., V. Beros, and Z. Klanfar, *Multiple cerebral aneurysms and a dural arteriovenous fistula in a patient with polyarteritis nodosa. Case illustration.* Journal of Neurosurgery, 2003. 98(2): p. 434.

[126] Ringer, A.J., L. Salud, and T.A. Tomsick, *Carotid cavernous fistulas: anatomy, classification, and treatment.* Neurosurgery Clinics of North America, 2005. 16(2): p. 279-95.

[127] Lasjaunias, P., *Lesion types, hemodynamics and clinical spectrum*, in *Dural arteriovenous malformations*, I. Awad and D. Barrow, Editors. 1993, AANS: Park Ridge, Illinois. p. 49-80.

[128] Sekhon, L.H., M.K. Morgan, and I.H. Johnston, *Syndactyly and intracranial arteriovenous malformation: case report.* British Journal of Neurosurgery, 1994. 8(3): p. 377-80.

[129] Friedman, A., *Etiologic factors in intracranial dural arteriovenous malformations*, in *Dural arteriovenous malformations*, I. Awad and D. Barrow, Editors. 1993, AANS: Park Ridge, Illinois. p. 35-48.

[130] Mullan, S., *Reflections upon the nature and management of intracranial and intraspinal vascular malformations and fistulae.* Journal of Neurosurgery, 1994. 80(4): p. 606-16.

[131] Klepach, G.L., et al., *Bilateral dural arteriovenous malformations simulating dysthyroid ophthalmopathy.* Annals of Ophthalmology, 1978. 10(11): p. 1519-23.

[132] Brown, R.D., Jr., D.O. Wiebers, and D.A. Nichols, *Intracranial dural arteriovenous fistulae: angiographic predictors of intracranial hemorrhage and clinical outcome in nonsurgical patients.* Journal of Neurosurgery, 1994. 81(4): p. 531-8.

[133] Houser, O.W., et al., *Intracranial dural arteriovenous malformations.* Radiology, 1972. 105(1): p. 55-64.

[134] Satomi, J., et al., *Benign cranial dural arteriovenous fistulas: outcome of conservative management based on the natural history of the lesion. [see comment].* Journal of Neurosurgery, 2002. 97(4): p. 767-70.

[135] Lasjaunias, P., C. Manelfe, and M. Chiu, *Angiographic architecture of intracranial vascular malformations and fistulas--pretherapeutic aspects.* Neurosurgical Review, 1986. 9(4): p. 253-63.

[136] Sundt, T.M., Jr. and D.G. Piepgras, *The surgical approach to arteriovenous malformations of the lateral and sigmoid dural sinuses.* Journal of Neurosurgery, 1983. 59(1): p. 32-9.

[137] Bederson, J., *Pathophysiology and animal models of dural arteriovenous malformations,* in *Dural arteriovenous malformations,* I. Awad and D. Barrow, Editors. 1993, AANS: Park Ridge, Illinois. p. 23-34.

[138] Kawaguchi, T., et al., *Hemodynamics before and after the total removal of a dural arteriovenous malformation of the posterior fossa. Case report.* Surgical Neurology, 1988. 30(6): p. 457-61.

[139] Kosnik, E.J., W.E. Hunt, and C.A. Miller, *Dural arteriovenous malformations.* Journal of Neurosurgery, 1974. 40(3): p. 322-9.

[140] Phelps, C.D., H.S. Thompson, and K.C. Ossoinig, *The diagnosis and prognosis of atypical carotid-cavernous fistula (red-eyed shunt syndrome).* American Journal of Ophthalmology, 1982. 93(4): p. 423-36.

[141] Grove, A.S., Jr., *The dural shunt syndrome. Pathophysiology and clinical course.* Ophthalmology, 1984. 91(1): p. 31-44.

[142] Lipton, R.B., et al., *Classification of primary headaches.* Neurology, 2004. 63(3): p. 427-35.

[143] Headache Classification Subcommittee of the International Headache, S., *The International Classification of Headache Disorders: 2nd edition.* Cephalalgia, 2004. 24 Suppl 1: p. 9-160.

[144] Heros, R.C. and J.J. Morcos, *Cerebrovascular surgery: past, present, and future.[see comment].* Neurosurgery, 2000. 47(5): p. 1007-33.

[145] Sarma, D. and K. ter Brugge, *Management of intracranial dural arteriovenous shunts in adults.* European Journal of Radiology, 2003. 46(3): p. 206-20.

[146] Awad, I., *Dural arteriovenous malformations with aggressive course,* in *Dural arteriovenous malformations,* I. Awad and D. Barrow, Editors. 1993, AANS: Park Ridge, Illinois. p. 93-104.

[147] Al-Mefty, O., J.R. Jinkins, and J.L. Fox, *Extensive dural arteriovenous malformation. Case report.* Journal of Neurosurgery, 1986. 65(3): p. 417-20.

[148] Lee, P.H., et al., *Parkinsonism as an initial manifestation of dural arteriovenous fistula.* European Journal of Neurology, 2005. 12(5): p. 403-6.

[149] Matsuda, S., et al., *Intracranial dural arteriovenous fistula (DAVF) presenting progressive dementia and parkinsonism.* Journal of the Neurological Sciences, 1999. 165(1): p. 43-7.

[150] Summers, P.E., J.M. Jarosz, and H. Markus, *MR angiography in cerebrovascular disease.* Clinical Radiology, 2001. 56(6): p. 437-56.

[151] Kendall, B. and I. Moseley, *Therapeutic embolisation of the external carotid arterial tree.* Journal of Neurology, Neurosurgery & Psychiatry, 1977. 40(10): p. 937-50.

[152] Halbach, V.V., et al., *Transvenous embolization of direct carotid cavernous fistulas.* Ajnr: American Journal of Neuroradiology, 1988. 9(4): p. 741-7.

[153] Pollock, B.E., et al., *Stereotactic radiosurgery and particulate embolization for cavernous sinus dural arteriovenous fistulae.* Neurosurgery, 1999. 45(3): p. 459-66; discussion 466-7.

[154] Link, M.J., et al., *The role of radiosurgery and particulate embolization in the treatment of dural arteriovenous fistulas.* Journal of Neurosurgery, 1996. 84(5): p. 804-9.

[155] Soderman, M., et al., *Gamma knife surgery for dural arteriovenous shunts: 25 years of experience.* J Neurosurg, 2006. 104(6): p. 867-75.

[156] Lewis, A.I., T.A. Tomsick, and J.M. Tew, Jr., *Management of tentorial dural arteriovenous malformations: transarterial embolization combined with stereotactic radiation or surgery.[see comment].* Journal of Neurosurgery, 1994. 81(6): p. 851-9.

[157] Pan, D.H., et al., *Stereotactic radiosurgery for the treatment of dural arteriovenous fistulas involving the transverse-sigmoid sinus.[see comment].* Journal of Neurosurgery, 2002. 96(5): p. 823-9.

[158] Aminoff, M.J., *Vascular anomalies in the intracranial dura mater.* Brain, 1973. 96(3): p. 601-12.

[159] Awad, I.A., et al., *Intracranial dural arteriovenous malformations: factors predisposing to an aggressive neurological course.* Journal of Neurosurgery, 1990. 72(6): p. 839-50.

[160] Borden, J.A., J.K. Wu, and W.A. Shucart, *A proposed classification for spinal and cranial dural arteriovenous fistulous malformations and implications for treatment.* Journal of Neurosurgery, 1995. 82(2): p. 166-79.

[161] Malik, G.M., et al., *Dural arteriovenous malformations and intracranial hemorrhage.* Neurosurgery, 1984. 15(3): p. 332-9.

[162] Davies, M., et al., *The natural history and management of intracranial dural arteriovenous fistulae. Part 2: aggressive lesions.* Interventional Neuroradiology, 1997. 3: p. 303-311.

[163] van Dijk, J.M., et al., *Clinical course of cranial dural arteriovenous fistulas with long-term persistent cortical venous reflux.* Stroke, 2002. 33(5): p. 1233-6.

[164] Duffau, H., et al., *Early rebleeding from intracranial dural arteriovenous fistulas: report of 20 cases and review of the literature.* Journal of Neurosurgery, 1999. 90(1): p. 78-84.

[165] Gautier, J.C., A. Awada, and P. Loron, *A cerebrovascular accident with unusual features.* Stroke, 1983. 14(5): p. 808-10.

[166] Hurst, R.W., et al., *Reversible arteriovenous malformation-induced venous hypertension as a cause of neurological deficits.* Neurosurgery, 1992. 30(3): p. 422-5.

[167] Hurst, R.W., et al., *Dementia resulting from dural arteriovenous fistulas: the pathologic findings of venous hypertensive encephalopathy.[see comment].* Ajnr: American Journal of Neuroradiology, 1998. 19(7): p. 1267-73.

[168] Ito, M., et al., *Reversible dural arteriovenous malformation-induced venous ischemia as a cause of dementia: treatment by surgical occlusion of draining dural sinus: case report.* Neurosurgery, 1995. 37(6): p. 1187-91; discussion 1191-2.

[169] Jaillard, A.S., B. Peres, and M. Hommel, *Neuropsychological features of dementia due to dural arteriovenous malformation.* Cerebrovascular Diseases, 1999. 9(2): p. 91-7.

[170] Katz, J.M., et al., *Transient aphasia and reversible major depression due to a giant sagittal sinus dural AV fistula.* Neurology, 2003. 61(4): p. 557-8.

[171] Tanaka, K., et al., *Dural arteriovenous malformation manifesting as dementia due to ischemia in bilateral thalami. A case report.* Surgical Neurology, 1999. 51(5): p. 489-93; discussion 493-4.

[172] Zeidman, S.M., et al., *Reversibility of white matter changes and dementia after treatment of dural fistulas.* Ajnr: American Journal of Neuroradiology, 1995. 16(5): p. 1080-3.

[173] Albuquerque, F.C., G.W. Heinz, and C.G. McDougall, *Reversal of blindness after transvenous embolization of a carotid-cavernous fistula: case report.* Neurosurgery, 2003. 52(1): p. 233-6; discussion 236-7.

[174] Brodsky, M.C., et al., *Recovery from total monocular blindness after balloon embolization of carotid-cavernous fistula.* American Journal of Ophthalmology, 1987. 104(1): p. 86-7.

[175] Davies, M., et al., *The natural history and management of intracranial dural arteriovenous fistulae. Part 1: benign lesions.* Interventional Neuroradiology, 1997. 3: p. 295-302.

[176] Friedman, J.A., et al., *Fatal progression of posttraumatic dural arteriovenous fistulas refractory to multimodal therapy. Case report.[see comment].* Journal of Neurosurgery, 2001. 94(5): p. 831-5.

[177] Klisch, J., et al., *Transvenous treatment of carotid cavernous and dural arteriovenous fistulae: results for 31 patients and review of the literature.* Neurosurgery, 2003. 53(4): p. 836-56; discussion 856-7.

[178] Kiyosue, H., et al., *Recurrence of dural arteriovenous fistula in another location after selective transvenous coil embolization: report of two cases.* Ajnr: American Journal of Neuroradiology, 2002. 23(4): p. 689-92.

[179] Kubo, M., et al., *Dural arteriovenous fistulae developing at different locations after resolution of previous fistulae: report of three cases and review of the literature.* Ajnr: American Journal of Neuroradiology, 2002. 23(5): p. 787-9.

[180] Sure, U., et al., *Endothelial proliferation, neoangiogenesis, and potential de novo generation of cerebrovascular malformations.* Journal of Neurosurgery, 2001. 94(6): p. 972-7.

[181] Raybaud, C.A., C.M. Strother, and J.K. Hald, *Aneurysms of the vein of Galen: embryonic considerations and anatomical features relating to the pathogenesis of the malformation.* Neuroradiology, 1989. 31(2): p. 109-28.

[182] Raybaud, C.A., et al., *Les anevrysmes de la veine de Galien. Etude angiographique et considerations morphogenetiques.* Neuro-Chirurgie, 1987. 33(4): p. 302-14.

[183] Yasargil, M., *Microneurosurgery IIIB.* Vol. IIIB. 1988, New York: Thieme.

[184] Lasjaunias, P., et al., *The role of dural anomalies in vein of Galen aneurysms: report of six cases and review of the literature.* Ajnr: American Journal of Neuroradiology, 1987. 8(2): p. 185-92.

[185] Halbach, V.V., et al., *Treatment of dural fistulas involving the deep cerebral venous system.* Ajnr: American Journal of Neuroradiology, 1989. 10(2): p. 393-9.

[186] Xu, D.S., et al., *Adult presentation of a familial-associated vein of galen aneurysmal malformation: case report.* Neurosurgery, 2010. 67(6): p. E1845-51; discussion 1851.

[187] Revencu, N., et al., *Parkes Weber syndrome, vein of Galen aneurysmal malformation, and other fast-flow vascular anomalies are caused by RASA1 mutations.* Hum Mutat, 2008. 29(7): p. 959-65.

[188] Lasjaunias, P., K. ter Brugge, and A. Berenstein, *Vein of Galen Aneurysmal Malformation,* in *Surgical Neuroangiography*2006, Springer: Berlin. p. 105-226.

[189] Hoang, S., et al., *Vein of Galen malformation.* Neurosurg Focus, 2009. 27(5): p. E8.

[190] Kalra, V. and A. Malhotra, *Fetal MR diagnosis of vein of Galen aneurysmal malformation.* Pediatr Radiol, 2010. 40 Suppl 1: p. S155.

[191] Brunelle, F., *Brain vascular malformations in the fetus: diagnosis and prognosis.* Childs Nerv Syst, 2003. 19(7-8): p. 524-8.

[192] Karadeniz, L., et al., *Vein of Galen aneurysmal malformation: prenatal diagnosis and early endovascular management.* J Chin Med Assoc, 2011. 74(3): p. 134-7.

[193] Khullar, D., A.M. Andeejani, and K.R. Bulsara, *Evolution of treatment options for vein of Galen malformations.* J Neurosurg Pediatr, 2010. 6(5): p. 444-51.

[194] Lasjaunias, P.L., et al., *The management of vein of Galen aneurysmal malformations.* Neurosurgery, 2006. 59(5 Suppl 3): p. S184-94; discussion S3-13.

[195] Payne, B.R., et al., *Gamma surgery for vein of Galen malformations.* J Neurosurg, 2000. 93(2): p. 229-36.

[196] Russell, D., L. Rubinstein, and C. Lumsden, *Tumors and hamartomas of the blood vessels,* in *Pathology of tumors of the nervous system,* D. Russell and L. Rubinstein, Editors. 1959, Edward Arnold: London. p. 72-92.

[197] McCormick, W.F., *The pathology of vascular ("arteriovenous") malformations.* J Neurosurg, 1966. 24(4): p. 807-16.

[198] Awad, I.A., et al., *Mixed vascular malformations of the brain: clinical and pathogenetic considerations.* Neurosurgery, 1993. 33(2): p. 179-88; discussion 188.

[199] Pozzati, E., et al., *The neurovascular triad: mixed cavernous, capillary, and venous malformations of the brainstem.* J Neurosurg, 2007. 107(6): p. 1113-9.

[200] Sayama, C.M., et al., *Capillary telangiectasias: clinical, radiographic, and histopathological features. Clinical article.* J Neurosurg, 2010. 113(4): p. 709-14.

[201] Scaglione, C., et al., *Symptomatic unruptured capillary telangiectasia of the brain stem: report of three cases and review of the literature.* J Neurol Neurosurg Psychiatry, 2001. 71(3): p. 390-3.

[202] Wijdicks, E.F. and W.I. Schievink, *Perimesencephalic nonaneurysmal subarachnoid hemorrhage: first hint of a cause?* Neurology, 1997. 49(2): p. 634-6.

[203] Umetsu, A., *MR imaging of vascular malformations,* in *Neurovascular Imaging,* S. Takahashi, Editor 2011, Springer-Verlag: London. p. 373-393.

[204] Tang, S.C., et al., *Diffuse capillary telangiectasia of the brain manifested as a slowly progressive course.* Cerebrovasc Dis, 2003. 15(1-2): p. 140-2.

[205] Huddle, D.C., J.C. Chaloupka, and V. Sehgal, *Clinically aggressive diffuse capillary telangiectasia of the brain stem: a clinical radiologic-pathologic case study.* AJNR Am J Neuroradiol, 1999. 20(9): p. 1674-7.

[206] Ruiz, D.S., H. Yilmaz, and P. Gailloud, *Cerebral developmental venous anomalies: current concepts.* Ann Neurol, 2009. 66(3): p. 271-83.

[207] Rammos, S.K., R. Maina, and G. Lanzino, *Developmental venous anomalies: current concepts and implications for management.* Neurosurgery, 2009. 65(1): p. 20-9; discussion 29-30.

[208] Kilic, T., et al., *Expression of structural proteins and angiogenic factors in cerebrovascular anomalies.* Neurosurgery, 2000. 46(5): p. 1179-91; discussion 1191-2.

[209] Lasjaunias, P., K. ter Brugge, and A. Berenstein, *Introduction and general comments regarding pediatric intracranial arteriovenous shunts,* in *Surgical Neuroangiography*2006, Springer: Berlin. p. 27-92.

[210] Saito, Y. and N. Kobayashi, *Cerebral venous angiomas: clinical evaluation and possible etiology.* Radiology, 1981. 139(1): p. 87-94.

[211] Wilson, C.B., *Cryptic vascular malformations.* Clin Neurosurg, 1992. 38: p. 49-84.

[212] Ruiz, D.S. and P. Gailloud, *Cerebral developmental venous anomalies.* Childs Nerv Syst, 2010. 26(10): p. 1395-1406.

[213] Abla, A., et al., *Developmental venous anomaly, cavernous malformation, and capillary telangiectasia: spectrum of a single disease.* Acta Neurochir (Wien), 2008. 150(5): p. 487-9; discussion 489.

[214] Ruiz, D.S.M., et al., *Parenchymal abnormalities associated with developmental venous anomalies.* Neuroradiology, 2007. 49(12): p. 987-95.

[215] Petersen, T.A., et al., *Familial versus sporadic cavernous malformations: differences in developmental venous anomaly association and lesion phenotype.* AJNR Am J Neuroradiol, 2010. 31(2): p. 377-82.

[216] Gandolfo, C., et al., *Sinus pericranii: diagnostic and therapeutic considerations in 15 patients.* Neuroradiology, 2007. 49(6): p. 505-14.

[217] Gabikian, P., et al., *Developmental venous anomalies and sinus pericranii in the blue rubber-bleb nevus syndrome. Case report.* J Neurosurg, 2003. 99(2): p. 409-11.

[218] Duffy, K., *Genetics and syndromes associated with vascular malformations.* Pediatr Clin North Am, 2010. 57(5): p. 1111-20.

[219] Brouillard, P. and M. Vikkula, *Genetic causes of vascular malformations.* Hum Mol Genet, 2007. 16 Spec No. 2: p. R140-9.

[220] Tan, W.H., et al., *The spectrum of vascular anomalies in patients with PTEN mutations: implications for diagnosis and management.* J Med Genet, 2007. 44(9): p. 594-602.

[221] McLaughlin, M.R., et al., *The prospective natural history of cerebral venous malformations.* Neurosurgery, 1998. 43(2): p. 195-200; discussion 200-1.

[222] Drummond, K.J., M.K. Morgan, and D.H. Brazier, *Intracranial haemorrhage associated with anomalous venous drainage.* J Clin Neurosci, 1998. 5(1): p. 87-90.

[223] Hanson, E.H., et al., *Developmental venous anomalies: appearance on whole-brain CT digital subtraction angiography and CT perfusion.* Neuroradiology, 2011. 53(5): p. 331-41.

[224] Fierstien, S.B., H.W. Pribram, and G. Hieshima, *Angiography and computed tomography in the evaluation of cerebral venous malformations.* Neuroradiology, 1979. 17(3): p. 137-48.

[225] Wurm, G., M. Schnizer, and F.A. Fellner, *Cerebral cavernous malformations associated with venous anomalies: surgical considerations.* Neurosurgery, 2005. 57(1 Suppl): p. 42-58; discussion 42-58.

[226] Sarwar, M. and W.F. McCormick, *Intracerebral venous angioma. Case report and review.* Arch Neurol, 1978. 35(5): p. 323-5.

[227] Washington, C.W., K.E. McCoy, and G.J. Zipfel, *Update on the natural history of cavernous malformations and factors predicting aggressive clinical presentation.* Neurosurg Focus, 2010. 29(3): p. E7.

[228] Stoodley MA and Weir BKA. *Aneurysms and arteriovenous malformations,* in *Diseases of the nervous system,* Asbury AK, McKhann GM, McDonald WI, Goadsby PJ, Editors 2002. Cambridge University Press, p 1392-1404.

[229] Tu J, Stoodley MA, Morgan MK, Storer KP. Ultrastructural characteristics of hemorrhagic, non-hemorrhagic and recurrent cavernous malformations. Journal of Neurosurgery 103:903-909, 2005.

[230] Kehrer-Sawatzki H, Wilda M, Braun VM, Richter HP, Hameister H. Mutation and expression analysis of the KRIT1 gene associated with cerebral cavernous malformations (CCM1). Acta Neuropathologica. 104(3):231-40, 2002.

[231] Zawistowski JS, Stalheim L, Uhlik MT, Abell AN, Ancrile BB, Johnson GL, Marchuk DA. CCM1 and CCM2 protein interactions in cell signaling: implications for cerebral cavernous malformations pathogenesis. Hum Mol Genet. 14(17):2521-31, 2005.

[232] Wurm G, Schnizer M, Nussbaumer K, Wies W, Holl K. Recurrent cryptic vascular malformation associated with a developmental venous anomaly. British Journal of Neurosurgery. 17(2):188-95, 2003.

[233] Abla AA. Lekovic GP. Garrett M. Wilson DA. Nakaji P. Bristol R. Spetzler RF. Cavernous malformations of the brainstem presenting in childhood: surgical experience in 40 patients. Neurosurgery 67:1589–1599, 2010.

4

Ultrasound Diagnosis of Congenital Brain Anomalies

Brankica Vasiljevic[1], Miroslava Gojnic[1] and Svjetlana Maglajlic-Djukic[2]
[1]*Institute of Gynecology and Obstetrics – Clinical Centre of Serbia,*
[2]*University Children's Hospital,*
Belgrade,
Serbia

1. Introduction

Congenital malformations affect approximately 2-3% of all live births every year (Whiteman et al, 1994; Atlas *et al*, 1985). Congenital brain anomalies, whether they are isolated (single) or part of syndromes, are a common cause of medical intervention, long-term illness, and death. The neonatologist or perinatologist often is the first person to identify necessary evaluations and management and to explain the cause of the anomalies and the prognosis for the child to the parents. Different anomalies may be classified as malformations, deformations and disruptions (Smith & Smith 2006; Barkovich *et al* 2001, Barkovich, 2005). Co-existent group of anomalies is described as polytopic field defect, sequence, syndrome and association. Other classification may be major and minor anomalies. Major anomaly is one with a medical, surgical or cosmetic importance and with impact on morbidity and mortality. Minor anomaly is one that does not have a serious surgical, medical or cosmetic significance and does not affect normal life expectancy or lifestyle.

Central nervous system (CNS) anomalies are the second most frequent serious congenital anomaly, after congenital heart disease. There is significant variation in incidences of congenital CNS anomalies in different regions of world including Europe (Barkovich, 2005). Congenital CNS anomalies are a heterogeneous disease for which genetic, infectious, teratogenic and neoplastic causes have been implicated (Bendon, 1987; Barkovich *et al*, 2005). Table 1. show the frequency of different CNS congenital anomalies which were detected in our institute during fourth years study period.

The development of the brain and spinal cord is an extremely complicated process which continues into second decade before final maturity is achieved. Abnormality in the development of CNS are common, up to 75 % of fetal deaths and 40% of deaths in infancy are due to CNS malformations (Barkovich, 2005). Furthermore, one third of all congenital abnormalities identified in the perinatal period arise from the central nervous system. These abnormalities are often evident at birth, but some cerebral malformations may not be immediately obvious. The neonates with dysmorphic feature or abnormal neurological behaviour may suggest cerebral malformations, and various imaging techniques are essential for further clarification. Due to the wide spectrum of congenital CNS abnormalities, only the more common ones amenable will be discussed here. Ultrasound (US) examination is an effective modality for the diagnosis of these anomalies in experienced hands. Cranial US correlate well with anatomical and pathological findings and clinical outcomes. Cranial US detection of congenital brain anomalies is useful for diagnostic purposes, and it also may allow for more appropriate management and more accurate neurological prognostication.

Congenital CNS anomalies	2005	2006	2007	2008	∑	Incidence
ACC	1			1	2	0.07 : 1000
Arachnoid cysts			1		1	0.03 : 1000
CSD	3	3	8	11	25	0.9 : 1000
DWM			1	1	2	0.07 : 1000
Encephaloceles		1			1	0.03 : 1000
Spinal lipoma			1		1	0.03 : 1000
Holoprosencephaly	2		1		3	0.1 : 1000
Hydrocephalus	9	2	1	4	15	0.5 : 1000
MCM				1	1	0.03 : 1000
Myelomeningoceles	4	1	5	2	12	0.4 : 1000
Microcephaly	1	1		1	3	0.1 : 1000
Schizencephaly				1	1	0.03 : 1000
VGA		1			1	0.03 : 1000
Ventriculomegaly	12	8	7	13	40	1.3 : 1000
Births	7091	7070	7015	7012	28818	3.6 : 1000

Table 1. The frequency of different CNS congenital anomalies (ACC- Agenesis of the corpus callosum; CSD- Closed spinal dysraphisms; DWM- Dandy-Walker malformation; MCM- Mega cistern magna; VGA-Vein of Galen aneurysm).

2. Cranial ultrasonography

In the neonatal period cranial US can be used as the initial modality to exclude a major structural malformation (Fawer, 1985; Carty *et al*, 2001, Barkovich, 2005; Von Wezel-Meijler G, 2007). Cranial ultrasonography (US) was introduced into neonatology in the late 1970s and has become an essential diagnostic tool in modern neonatology. It is non-invasive highly sensitive, safe, easily repeatable, accurate and cost effective neuroimaging technique. The advantages of cranial US are that it can be performed at the bedside with minimal disturbance to the neonates and patients do not require sedation. It is a useful modality for detecting congenital and acquired anomalies of the brain and the most frequently occurring patterns of brain injury in both preterm and full-term neonates. Cranial US is also suitable for assessing brain maturation and timing of cerebral injury. It can be initiated at a very early stage, even immediately after birth. Cranial US is relatively inexpensive compared with other neuro-imaging techniques. The non-invasive nature of cranial US make it an ideal imaging technique in the neonate. During the late foetal and perinatal period and during early infancy, major maturational processes and growth of the brain take place

(Barkovich *et al*, 2001; Carty *et al* 2001). Maturational processes include a major increase in volume, weight, and surface area of the brain; gyration; cell migration; germinal matrix involution; and myelination. These maturation processes can be visualised by modern neuro-imaging techniques. Gyration is a phenomenon occurring late during fetal development and can be observed by the second month of intrauterine life. It goes on to the end of the pregnancy and even later after birth. The primary sulci appear as shallow grooves on the surface of the brain that become progressively more deeply infolded and that develop side branches, designated secondary sulci. Gyration proceeds with the formation of other side branches of the secondary sulci, referred to as tertiary sulci. The timing of the appearance of these different types of sulci is so precise that neuropathologists consider gyration to be a reliable estimate of gestational age and consequently a good marker of fetal brain maturation (Figure 1.).

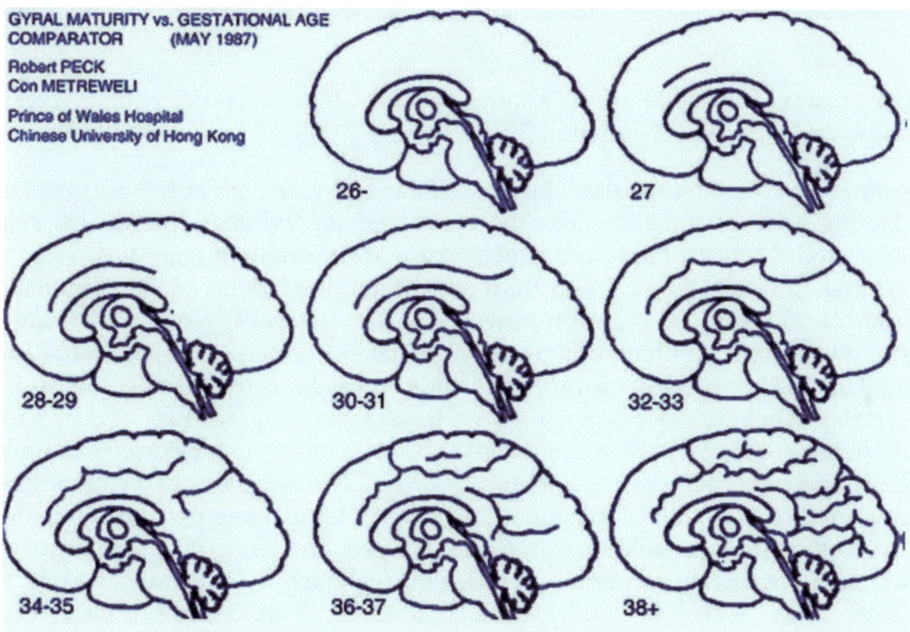

Fig. 1. Comparative sagittal sections show a gyral pattern from 26-38+ weeks of gestation.

It is possible to assess the gestation age of the infant from the ultrasound images (Figure.2.). In extremely preterm infants (gestation age from 24–26 weeks), the brain surface is still very smooth and has a lissencephalic appearance. The process of gyration can be followed by cranial US and cortical sulcation is considered to be a good marker of neonatal brain maturation by neuropathologists (Barkovich, 2005; Von Wezel-Meijler, 2007). Familiarity with the normal ultrasonographic imaging appearances of the fetal/neonatal cerebral cortex at various stages of gestation is essential for the early detection of abnormal sulcal development. Abnormal cortical development is the main manifestation of lissencephaly, although other associated CNS anomalies (e.g. ventriculomegaly, holoprosencephaly, agenesis of the corpus callosum, porencephaly, encephalocele).

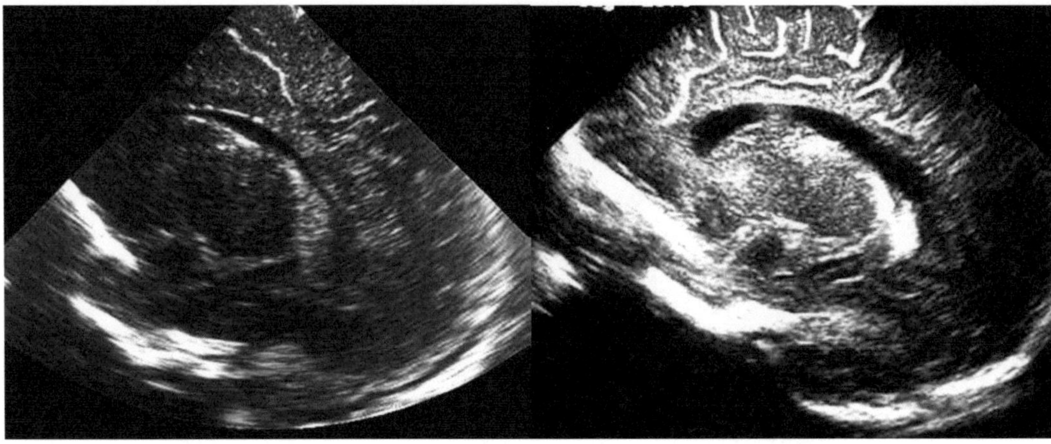

a b

Fig. 2. Comparative US sagittal sections show a gyral pattern in neonate with 27 weeks of gestation (A) and 38 weeks of gestation (B).

The germinal matrix is an abundant, highly cellular and vascular "strip" of subependymal tissue. During early gestation it lines the entire wall of the lateral ventricles and third ventricle. It produces neuroblasts and glioblasts and is the origin of migrating neurons (first trimester) and glial cells (second and third trimesters). Regression of the germinal matrix starts from 24–26 weeks of gestation onwards. After 34 weeks, remnants remain in the thalamo-caudate notch and temporal horns of the lateral ventricles. In the foetus and very preterm infant, the lateral ventricles are often wide and asymmetric (usually the left is larger than the right) with very wide occipital horns. Subarachnoid spaces may also be wide. The cerebral lateral ventricles have a complex threedimensional architecture that undergoes major developmental changes throughout gestation. Normal sizes of ventricles provide reassurance of the normal development of the neonatal brain. Lateral ventricles are slightly, but significantly, larger in male than in female fetuses. Therefore, it is not surprising that males are found to have borderline ventriculomegaly more frequently, and to have a significantly lesser degree of neurological compromise than females (Pilu *et al*, 1999). Spontaneous remission of borderline ventriculomegaly is frequently documented. It is unclear whether or not this implies an amelioration of the prognosis. Some investigators failed to demonstrate a difference in the outcome between cases with stable or progressing ventriculomegaly and cases with spontaneous remission (Pilu *et al*, 1999). Mild ventriculomegaly may be the first sign of abnormal or delayed brain maturation. It is possible that isolated borderline ventriculomegaly may represent the earliest manifestation of brain damage from heterogeneous causes including primary cerebral maldevelopment (e.g. obstructive hydrocephalus, lissencephaly) and destructive lesions (e.g. periventricular leukomalacia) arising from hypoxia and/or infections. Gross enlargement consistently indicates major cerebral anomalies.

Standard cranial US scanning is performed through the anterior fontanel, the whole brain is scanned, and images are recorded in at least six coronal and five sagittal planes with a high frequency sector transducer (7.5-10 MHz). These imaging planes are shown in Figure 3.

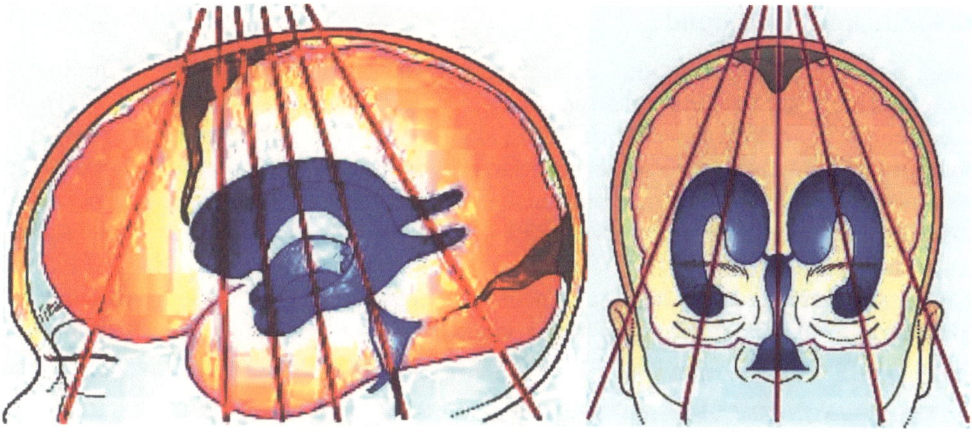

a b

Fig. 3. Technique of intracranial scanning: (A) coronal planes; (B) sagittal planes.

An additional scan series can be obtained in the axial plane through the temporoparietal bone. The standard coronal and sagittal views are used to assess the symmetry of the cerebral hemispheres, absence of the CSP and the corpus callosum, morphology of the cerebral ventricles, thalami and the posterior cranial fossa structures (e.g. cerebellum, the cisterna magna and the fourth ventricle). A high frequency linear transducer (10 MHz) is very useful to examine the subarachnoid and subdural space and integrity of the spine (Figure 4.a.). Doppler is extremely useful for the routine cranial examination. This is particularly true when trying to differentiate subdural from subarachnoid fluid in the subarachnoid spaces (Figure 4.b.) and in any suspected vascular lesion such as a vein of Galen anomaly (Chavhan *et al*, 2008). Cranial US are correlated with anatomical and pathological findings and clinical outcomes. Appropriate correlation of the US features with clinical history can assist in improving the diagnostic yield. Familiarity with the US features of congenital brain anomalies is therefore an extremely valuable tool, as it facilitates an accurate diagnosis and treatment these anomalies.

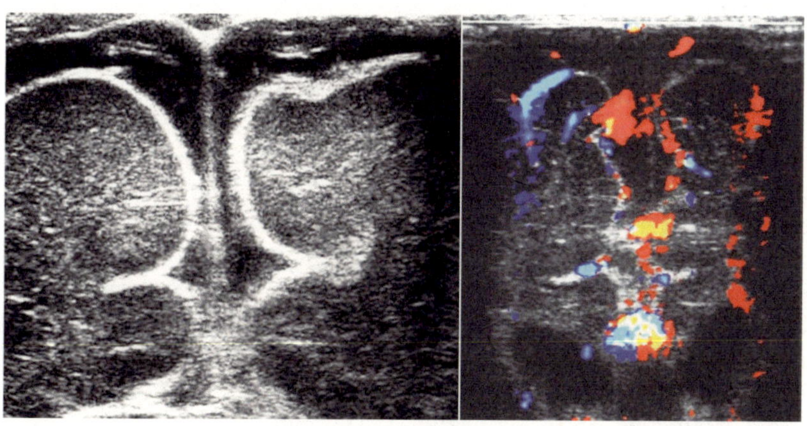

a b

Fig. 4. Normal surface subdural and subarachnoid spaces in coronal view using a high frequency linear transducer (A) and color Doppler (B).

2.1 Color doppler ultrasound

The use of pulsed and continuous color Doppler US allows simultaneous examination of parenchymal and vascular cerebral structures (Cheung *et al*, 1994; Vasiljevic *et al*, 2011). Pulsed and continuous color Doppler neuroimaging are used to assess cerebral blood flow in many pathological states including hypoxic ischemic change and congenital abnormalities. Doppler flow measurements may help to distinguish between vascular structures and non-vascular lesions. Cerebral blood flow accounts for 22%–25% of the cardiac output in neonates and 15% of that in adults (Couture, 2001). Every major vessel in the human body has a characteristic flow pattern that is visible in spectral waveforms obtained in that vessel with Doppler US. Familiarity with the Doppler waveforms characteristic of cerebral arteries and veins in neonates is important for accurate diagnosis of brain abnormalities (Figure 5.).

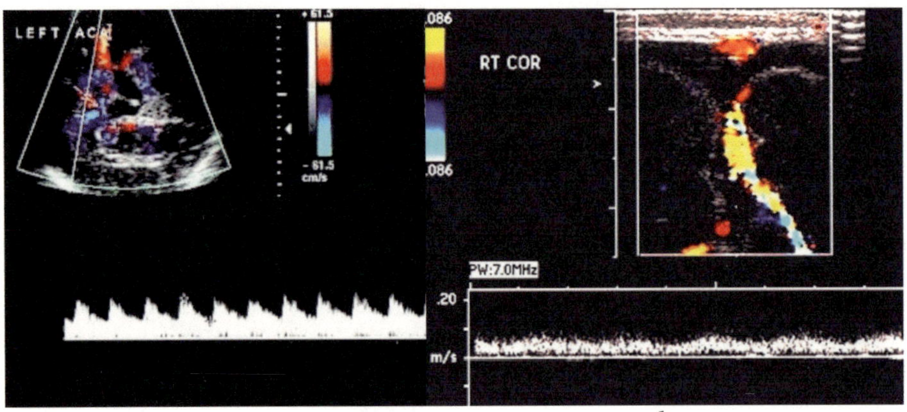

a b

Fig. 5. Normal color Doppler wave forms from the anterior cerebral artery (A) and the superior sagittal sinus (B).

The wave forms may be affected by age- and development-related hemodynamic differences (Chavhan *et al*, 2008, Romagnol *et al*, 2006). Values of cerebral blood flow velocities progressive increase with gestation age on consequence of progressive increase cardiac output, blood pressure and closing ductus arterosus (Vasiljevic *et al*, 2010). Values of Doppler indices (Pourcelot index or the resistance index and Gossling index or the pulsatility index) gradually increase with gestation age in consequence of progressive maturation and opening of vascular cerebral bed with a reduction of the cerebrovascular resistance (Vasiljevic *et al*, 2008; Deeg & Rupprecht, 1988). In the first 2 or 3 months after birth, complex variations in cerebral hemodynamics occur in association with changes in pO_2, pCO_2, and ductus arteriosus closure. Vasodilatation is seen with hypoxemia and hypercapnea. After the 3rd day of life, there is a gradual increase in peak systolic velocity and end-diastolic velocity. All cerebral arteries display a low-resistance flow pattern with continuous forward flow during systole and diastole (Figure 5.a.). Because these arteries usually have a diameter of less than 5 mm, the spectral lines are broad and the spectral window is filled. Knowledge of normal values of cerebral blood flow velocities and Doppler indices in neonates different gestation age is important for the monitoring maturational processes and growth of the immature brain and also useful for differential diagnosis of congenital and acquired CNS anomalies in both preterm and full-term neonates (Chavhan *et al,* 2008;). Normal neonatal values and postnatal changes of cerebral blood flow velocities have been reported by several examiners (Deeg & Rupprecht 1989; Romagnol *et al,* 2006; Vasiljevic *et al,* 2010). Table 2. shows the normal values of cerebral blood flow velocities and 3 Doppler indices in the anterior cerebral artery in neonates different gestation age. These values we have obtained with color Doppler technique in seventy healthy neonates different gestation age during two years study period.

Neonates	GA	BW (g)	PSV (cm/s)	EDV (cm/s)	RI	PI
10	27.3±0.5	950±110	21.30 ±0.45	6.40±0.20	0.59±0.10	1.06±0.08
20	29.5±1.2	1350±170	24.20 ±0.65	7.00±0.30	0.60±0.10	1.10±0.15
20	34.5±0.6	1950±340	27.00 ±0.75	7.80±0.50	0.63±0.08	1.15±0.30
20	38.6±1.3	3540±640	32.50 ±0.90	9.95±0.40	0.65±0.05	1.18±0.35
Σ 70	34.5± 5.5	2540 ±950	26.25±0.68	7.78±0.35	0.61±0.08	1.12±0.22

Table 2. Normal values of cerebral blood low velocities in the neonates in the neonates (GA- gestational age; PSV- peak-systolic velocity; EDV- end-diastolic velocity; RI- resistive index and PI- pulsatility index).

Referred cardiac pulsations normally can be seen in the intracranial veins. Venous waveforms in the superior sagittal sinus may be continuous and monophasic or may fluctuate in synchronicity with arterial pulsations (Figure 5.b.). Intracranial venous flow velocities gradually increase after birth (Dean & Taylor, 1995). The mean velocity in the superior sagittal sinus usually ranges between 8 and 12 cm/s in neonates. The transverse sinus usually can be assessed in neonates and shows an intracranial venous flow velocity of 2.7–3.3 cm/s. However, great variations can be seen in flow velocity with factors such as head rotation, crying, and other activities. Cardiac output fluctuates in an unstable neonate, altering carotid artery and cerebral perfusion. Color Doppler imaging is also useful in defining the limit of the arterial system within the subarachnoid space. This helps differentiate fluid in the subdural space from adhesions within the arachnoid space, as the arterial system is confined to the subarachnoid space (Chavhan *et al,* 2008; Dean & Taylor, 1995)

2.2 Ultrasnography of the spine

Ultrasound does not penetrate through bone but in the neonate the posterior spinal arches are poorly mineralized, allowing US assessment of the cord and dural sac from the foramen magnum down to the sacral hiatus. Spinal US is used as an initial screening tool in the neonate with spinal and other congenital abnormalities. There is a high incidence of spinal abnormalities in babies who have other congenital syndromes (e.g., ano-rectal malformation, cloacal exstrophy, caudal regression and spinal segmentation abnormalities—the VATER/VACTEROL anomaly) (Pilu & Hobbins, 2002). Two types of scanning planes can be used to evaluate the integrity of the spine. In transverse planes or axial planes, the examination of the spine is a dynamic process performed by sweeping the transducer along the entire length of the spine and at the same time keeping in the axial plane of the level being examined. In transverse sections, the neural canal appears as a closed circle. It is lined anteriorly by the ossification center in the body of the vertebrae and posteriorly by the two ossification centers of the laminae (Figure 6.). The vertebrae have different anatomic configurations at different levels. Thoracic and lumbar vertebrae have a triangular shape, while the first cervical vertebrae are quadrangular in shape, and sacral vertebrae are flat. In the longitudinal or saggital section, the spine appears as three parallel lines converging caudally in the sacrum. The lines correspond to the anterior and posterior walls of the spinal cord and a central echogenic line the central canal (Figure 6.). Spinal cord appears hypo-echoic. The cord is surrounded by the cerebrospinal fluid (CSF) which appears anechoic. In term neonates the conus medullaris is usually found at the level of L2-L3. If a true longitudinal section can be obtained, visualizing the conus medullaris in its normal location further strengthens the diagnosis of normalcy (Robbin *et al*, 1994). The filum terminale extends to the sacral region as a thin extension of the cord. The normal filum terminale is 1.0-1.5 mm in diameter. Filing the cord in this area are echogenic lines, nerve fibres, which almost fill the arachnoid space and can be seen to move on real-time imagining and form cauda eqina.

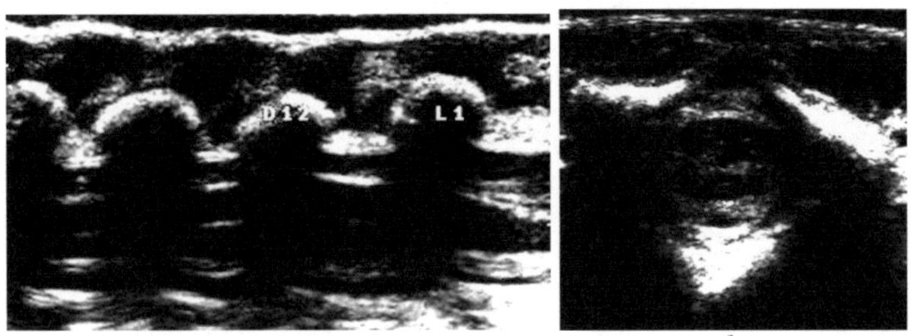

a b

Fig. 6. The longitudinal section of the neonatal spine (A) and the transverse views of the neonatal spine (B).

More recently three-dimensional ultrasound has become available. Three-dimensional ultrasound may facilitate the examination of the fetal brain and spine.

Its utility in the neonatal nursery needs further assessment, but it may be useful in assessing ventricular volumes and producing more meaningful images of cerebral abnormalities and brain damage (Riccabona *et al*, 2003). The main indication for MRI of the neonatal brain is further evaluation of inconclusive ultrasound findings in neonates with dysmorphic feature or abnormal neurological behavior.

3. Cerebral ventriculomegaly and hydrocephaly

Hydrocephalus and ventriculomegaly are both terms used to describe dilatation of the lateral ventricles. However, they should be distinguished: hydrocephalus signifies dilated lateral ventricles resulting from an increased amount of CSF inside the ventricles and increased intracranial pressure, while ventriculomegaly is a dilatation of the lateral ventricles without increased intracranial, from any cause, nonobstructive or obstructive. Ventriculomegaly is the most common congenital CNS anomaly with an incidence of 0.3 to 1.5 per 1000 births, probably higher in utero (Fransen *et al*, 1996). Couples with a previously affected child have a recurrence risk of 4% (Griffiths *et al*, 2006). Ventriculomegaly can be isolated or associated with other congenital (e.g. Dandy Walker malformation, corpus callosum agenesis, arachnoid cysts, vein of Galen aneurysms and a spinal defect with myelomeningocele) or acquired CNS anomalies (hemorrhage, infections). Extra-cranial abnormalities occur in 30% of cases and included meningomyelocele, renal anomalies (e.g. bilateral or unilateral renal agenesis, dysplastic kidneys), cardiac anomalies (e.g. ventricular septal defect, tetralogy of Fallot), gastrointestinal anomalies (e.g. colon and anal agenesis, malrotation of the bowel), cleft lip and palate, Meckel syndrome, gonadal dysgenesis, arthrogryposis, and dysplastic phalanges. Chromosomal aberrations are found in 11% of cases, mostly trisomy 21 (Schwanitz *et al,* 1993; Gaglioti *et al,* 2005). Isolated congenital ventriculomegaly accounts for 30-60% of neonates with enlarged lateral cerebral ventricles (Mercier *et al,* 2001). In the majority of cases, isolated ventriculomegaly is the consequence of an obstruction along the normal pathway of CSF (e.g. obstructive ventriculomegaly). Nonobstructive causes of ventriculomegaly include a congenital CNS malformation (failure of development of portions of the normal brain), brain destruction (e.g. congenital infection or a vascular mechanism) and overproduction of CSF (choroid plexus papillomas). Congenital ventriculomegaly is a heterogeneous disease for which genetic, infectious, teratogenic and neoplastic causes have been implicated. A multifactorial pattern of inheritance is probably responsible for most cases of congenital ventriculomegaly (Renier *et al,* 1988). X-linked hydrocephalus comprises approximately 5% of all cases. This condition is caused by mutations in the gene at Xq28 encoding for L1, a neural cell adhesion molecule. Mutations in this gene are also responsible for other syndromes with clinical overlap that are frequently referred to as the X-linked hydrocephalus spectrum and include MASA (e.g. mental retardation, aphasia, shuffling gait, adducted thumbs) syndrome, X-linked mental retardation-clasped thumb (MR-CT) syndrome, X-linked complicated spastic paraparesis (SP1), and some forms of X-linked agenesis of the corpus callosum (Kenwick *et al,* 1996). The presence of uni- or bilateral ventriculomegaly seems to be of some discriminatory value. Ventriculomegaly tends to be unilateral in cases of brain destruction and bilateral in cases of CNS malformation, and this difference is statistically significant. In apparently isolated ventriculomegaly, we must distinguish between borderline and moderate to severe ventriculomegaly (Graham *et al,* 2001; Toma & Granata, 2005). US is an effective mode for imaging the ventricular system and sensitive to ventricular dilatation and minor degrees of ventricular asymmetry (Kenwick *et al,* 1996). In the clinically normal term infant the ventricles are often small (slit-like) for the few days after vaginal delivery. The normal ventricular system, which appears as anechogenic fluid-filled space becomes dilated and increase in size (Figure 7.).

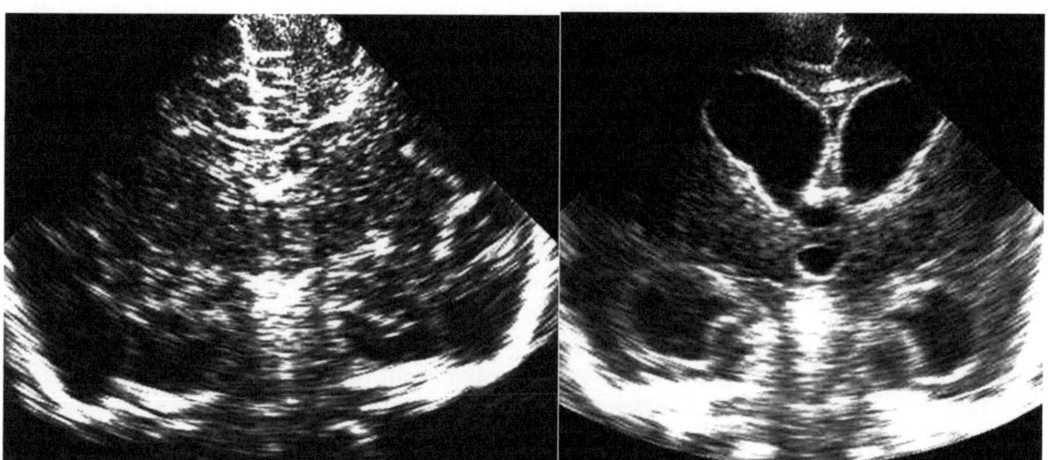

a b

Fig. 7. Normal ventricular system (A) and ventricular dilatation (B) in coronal view.

The most useful qualitative US features of early ventricular dilatation are ballooning of the supratentorial angles of the ventricles of the frontal horns in coronal plane. These areas dilate more than the trigones and bodies of the ventricles because they are lager and require less pressure for distension (Carty *et al*, 2001). Despite that, ventricular dilatation is usually first seen in the occipital horns of the lateral ventricles, but there is considerable variation in the size of this part of the ventricular system in normal babies. With modern real-time ultrasound, clear visualisation of the lateral ventricles can be obtained and exact anatomical landmarks identified. Lateral ventricular size has been measured with number of different methods. Levine et al measured the ventricular size from midline to the lateral-most point of the lateral ventricles (ventricular index) in 273 infant from 26 to 42week's gestation and described normal ranges of ventricular size at differing gestation (Levine *et al*, 1985). In addition, London et al measured the biventricular diameter at the level of the frontal horns, diagonal width of the frontal horns at level of the caudate nucleus, intercaudate distance and biventricular diameter at the body of the lateral ventricles (London *et al*, 1980). Allan et al and Qusling et al measured of the lateral ventricules at the mid-body near the atrium of ventricule in sagittal plane (Qusling yet al, 1983). This is regarded as a "standard table" for assessment of ventricular dilatation. The term borderline ventriculomegaly is commonly used to indicate cases characterized by an atrial width of 10–15 mm. Some authors have reported a different rate of abnormal neurologic outcome in fetuses with atria > 12 mm compared with those with atria measuring 10–12 mm (a mild form of borderline ventriculomegaly). In fact, an isolated borderline ventriculomegaly of 10–12 mm might be considered as a variant of the norm (Signorelli et al, 2004). When the atrial width is between 15–20 mm the ventriculomegaly is defined moderate. Aqueductal stenosis, regardless of its cause, is responsible for the progression of ventricular dilatation. Severe ventriculomegaly is usually referred to as hydrocephalus and is defined on the basis of an atrial width of more than 20 mm (Bloom *et al*, 1997) (Figure 7.b.). Congenital hydrocephalus is classified into three categories by causes that disturb the CSF circulation pathway: simple hydrocephalus, dysgenetic hydrocephalus, and secondary hydrocephalus. Simple hydrocephalus is caused by a developmental abnormality localized within the CSF circulation pathway and includes aqueductal stenosis, atresia of the foramen of Monro, Magendie or Luschka, and maldevelopment of arachnoid granulation. Dysgenetic hydrocephalus results from a cerebral developmental disorder in the early stages of development, and includes hydranencephaly, holoprosencephaly, porencephaly, schizencephaly, Dandy-Walker malformation, dysraphism, and Chiari malformation. Secondary hydrocephalus is a generic term indicating hydrocephalus caused by an intracranial pathologic condition, such as intracranial infection, hemorrhage or brain tumor.

Pediatric data suggest that a correlation exists between cortical mantle thickness before shunting and long-term intellectual performances. Thickness of less than 1 cm has been associated with a poor outcome, but the most important prognostic consideration is the presence and nature of the associated anomalies. The available evidence suggests that borderline ventriculomegaly is most frequently without consequences (Bloom *et al*, 1997). Some authors have opposite results, and suggest that borderline ventriculomegaly carries an increased risk of cerebral maldevelopment, delayed neurologic development, and possibly chromosomal aberrations (Pilu Falco *et al*, 1999; Mercier *et al*, 2001). The main problem in these cases with borderline ventriculomegaly is to exclude other CNS and extra-cranial malformations. Macrocrania at birth, ventricular size and age at surgery had no influence on the outcome. Ventriculomegaly may develop in late gestation or after birth, particularly with the X-linked hydrocephalus spectrum.

4. Agenesis of the corpus callosum

Agenesis of the corpus callosum is an anomaly that may occur in isolation or in association with other CNS or systemic malformations. Because the corpus callosum may be partially or completely absent, the term dysgenesis has also been used to describe the spectrum of callosal anomalies (Barkovich & Norman, 1988; Davila-Gutierrez, 2002). With complete agenesis, the corpus callosum is totally absent. With partial agenesis (hypoplasia), the anterior portion (posterior genu and anterior body) is formed, but the posterior portion (posterior body and splenium) is not. An atypical appearance occurs when the anterior to posterior formation is not respected (Barkovich, 1990). Development the corpus callosum occurs at the same time as cerebral and cerebellar development, and therefore agenesis of the corpus callosum is associated with other brain anomalies in 80% of cases. Associated CNS anomalies may include midline intracerebral lipomas, encephalocele, interhemispheric arachnoid cyst, microcephaly, Dandy-Walker malformation, Arnold-Chiari malformation, holoprosencephaly, hydrocephalus, disorders of neuronal migration, such as neuronal heterotopias, lissencephaly, pachygyria, and schizencephaly (Hetts *et al*, 2006; Volpe, 2009). With partial agenesis (hypogenesis), the anterior portion (posterior genu and anterior body) is formed, but the posterior portion (posterior body and splenium) is not. The rostrum and the anterior/inferior genu are also not formed. Secondary destruction of the corpus callosum occurs when the genu and anterior body are destroyed, leaving the posterior portion of the corpus callosum intact. Primary dysgenesis/agenesis of the corpus callosum should be differentiated from secondary destruction of an initially normally developed corpus callosum as can be observed in trauma, infarction, hemorrhage and in several metabolic diseases. Agenesis of the corpus callosum can occur in chromosomal abnormalities, such as trisomy 8, trisomy 13 and trisomy 18, as a part of the holoprosencephalic sequence, and also may be found in chromosomal translocation syndromes (Tang *et al*, 2009). Callosal anomalies are found in several syndromes, including X-linked Aicardi syndrome, the median cleft face syndrome, Andermann syndrome, F.G. syndrome, and acrocallosal syndrome. An association with maternal rubella and toxoplasmosis has been reported. Because they develop embryonically in close proximity, agenesis of the corpus callosum is commonly associated with malformations of local limbic structures, particularly the septum and hippocampal formations. Extra-CNS malformations may include anomalies of the face, musculoskeletal system, gastrointestinal tract, genitourinary tract, cardiovascular system, and respiratory system.

The incidence of agenesis of the corpus callosum is from 0.3–0.7% in the general population to 2–3% in the developmentally disabled population. Dependent on etiology, a recurrence risk is from 1% (if sporadic or chromosomal) to 25% (if autosomal recessive) or even 50% in males (if X-linked recessive).

The corpus callosum is a white matter structure connecting the cerebral hemispheres and is important in coordinating information and bilateral exchange of sensory stimuli. It develops between the 10th and 20th weeks of gestation, from the lamina reuniens, which is the thickened dorsal aspect of the lamina terminalis (Bennet *et al*, 1996). If the commissural plate fails to develop or is damaged, the uncrossed callosal fibers run parallel to the medial walls of the lateral ventricles, forming the bundles of Probst. These bundles do not cross the midline. Pathogenesis agenesis of the corpus callosum is uncertain, but callosal dysgenesis may be associated with a migration disorder (Smith *et al*, 2008). When complete, corpus callosum consist of genu, body, splenum and rostrum. The normal development sequence is anterior to posterior, which allows one to distinguish between a partial primary and secondary dysgenesis of the corpus callosum. The genu is the first area to develop. Antenatal diagnosis of agenesis of the corpus callosum is possible from about 20 weeks' gestation.

The characteristic findings agenesis of the corpus callosum on ultasonography included absent corpus callosum and cavum pellucidum in coronal and saggital planes, widely separated lateral venticles, colpocephaly or "teardrop" configuration of lateral ventricles, elevation and variable dilatation of the third ventricle ("interhemispheric cyst"), distended interhemispheric fissure, abnormal radial orientation of medial cerebral gyri extending from the roof of the third ventricle ("sunburst sign") and abnormal branching of anterior cerebral artery (Figure 8.) (Penny, 2006; Atlas *et al*, 1985; Byrd *et al*, 1990).

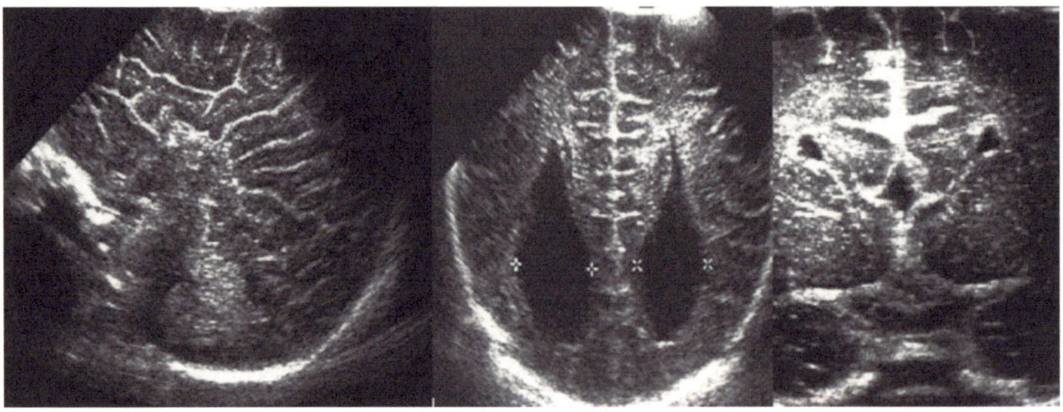

a b c

Fig. 8. Agenesis of the corpus callosum in the sagittal planes (A) and coronal planes; (B and C).

Color Doppler scan showing the absence of the corpus callosum and abnormal course of the pericallosal artery (Figure 9.). (Schell-Apacik *et al,* 2008). Lipoma of the corpus callosum is demonstrated as a highly echogenic mass in the region of the corpus callosum.

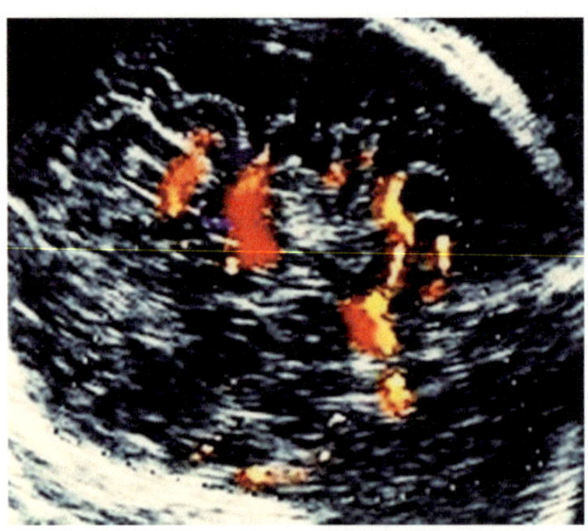

Fig. 9. Sagittal color Doppler scan shows the agenesis of the corpus callosum.

Agenesis of the corpus callosum may be a completely asymptomatic (found incidentally) or with subtle developmental deficits and severe neurologic problems, such as seizures, intellectual impairment, and psychosis. However, these conditions are believed to be caused by abnormalities in associated cerebral and chromosomal anomalies rather than in the corpus callosum per se (Goodyear *et al*, 2001). Hence, prognosis is determined primarily by the underlying or associated malformations. Studies of persons with isolated agenesis of the corpus callosum without other abnormalities show that some have normal intelligence, while others are developmentally delayed (Taylor *et al*, 1998). Complete agenesis has a worse prognosis than partial agenesis.

5. Holoprosencephaly

Holoprosencephaly is a heterogeneous entity of CNS anomalies caused by the impaired midline cleavage of the forebrain (prosencephalon) into the right and left hemispheres, and the malformation of the diencephalon, telencephalon, olfactory, and optic bulbs (Volpe, 2001).

Holoprosencephaly is graded according to the severity of the brains anomaly as alobar, semilobar and lobar (Figure 10.)(Peebles, 2001).

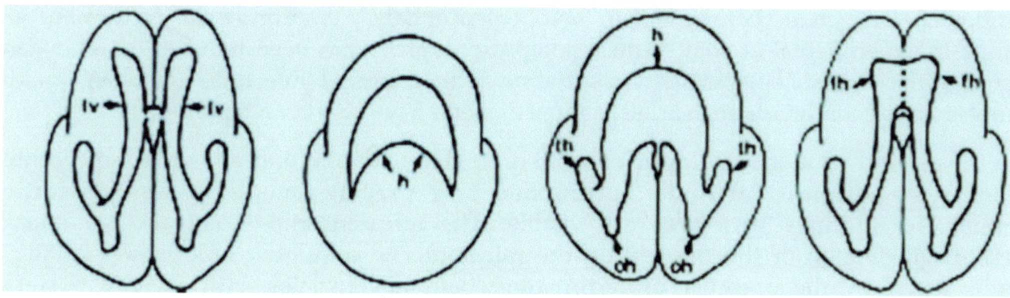

a b c d

Fig. 10. Schematic drawing of the normal neonatal brain (A), alobar holoprosencephaly (B), semilobar holoprosencephaly (C) and. lobar holoprosencephaly (D).

In alobar holoprosencephaly, the most severe form, the cerebral hemispheres are fused and enclose a single prosencephalic ventricle. There is a complete failure of cleavage of the forebrain into two hemispheres. It results in a single ventricular cavity with fusion of thalami, absence of corpus callosus, falx cerebri, optic tracts and olfactory bulbs. Partial cleavage results in semilobar holoprosencephaly, with posterior separation of the cerebral hemispheres, variable degrees of fusion of the thalami and absent olfactory bulbs and corpus callosus. In lobar holoprosencephaly, the abnormalities may be confined to absence of the corpus callosus and fusion of the lateral ventricles and cingulate gyrus. The two hemispheres are separated anteriorly and posteriorly. Because of a mechanism of reciprocal induction between the brain and the skull, the facial structures are also abnormal (Edison & Muenke, 2003). The severity of the facial malformation reflects the severity of the intracranial anomalies and include: cyclopia (median monoophthalmia, synophthalmia or anophthalmia with proboscis), cebocephaly or« monkey head », (ocular hypotelorism and a blind single nostril nose), ethmocephaly (ocular hypotelorism with proboscis) and median cleft lip.

Holoprosencephaly is found in several syndromes, including Meckel-Gruber syndrome, holoprosencephaly-fetal akinesia syndrome and Steinfield syndrome (Cho *et al*, 2005). The most frequently associated CNS anomalies are microcephaly, macrocephaly, and Dandy-Walker malformations. Associated extra-cranial abnormalities are congenital heart defects, renal dysplasias, omphalocele and polydactyly.

The incidence holoprosencephaly is about to 0.6-1.9 per 1000 births, but 4 per 1000 in embryos. Half of these are associated with trisomy 13. Holoprosencephaly occurs in about 70% of the patients with trisomy 13 (Roessler & Muenke, 1998). The sex distribution shows a female predominance. The risk of recurrence depends of the basis for the actual condition, such as chromosome defect or syndrome. In the cases without chromosomal abnormalities, the recurrence risk is estimated to be 6%.

The etiology of holoprosencephaly is heterogeneous and not completely known. Most cases are sporadic and environmental, and genetic factors have all been implicated as possible causes (Muenke & Beachey, 2000). This is probably due to mutations in the gene for the sonic hedgehog morphogen and genes that encode its downstream intracellular signaling pathway (Wallis & Muenke, 2000). There is also some evidence for a defect in the cholesterol biosynthesis. Holoprosencephaly in association with extra cephalic malformations suggests aneuploidy, particularly trisomy 13. Familial holoprosencephaly is known. It can be inherited in an autosomal dominant fashion with varied penetrance, or as an autosomal recessive. In addition to the genetic component to holoprosencephaly , environmental factors are also critical. In experimental animal studies, holoprosencephaly has been induced by teratogenic agents (retinoic acid, ethanol). An association with maternal infectious (cytomegalovirus, toxoplasmosis), conditions such as gestational diabetes have also been reported.

The ultrasound of alobar holoprosencephaly is characteristic and shows a large central echo-free monoventricular cavity surrounded by a varying amount of residual cortical mantle. No midlines structures are visible. The infratentorial structures are usually present with fusion of the thalami on the midline. The semilobar holoprosencephaly is characterized by the presence of rudimentary lateral ventricles with sketchy posterior horns, and a more developed cortex, partial development of the interhemispheric fissure and of the falx cerebri, which is present only posteriorly and partial fusion of the thalami (Figure 11.). The lobar holoprosencephaly has a well developed interhemispheric fissure, partial fusion of the frontal horns with the third ventricle, hypoagenesis of the corpus callosum and the cavum septum pellucidum is absent.

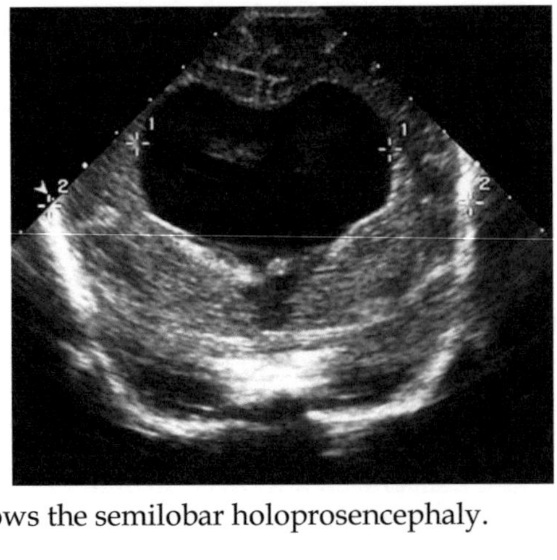

Fig. 11. Coronal scan shows the semilobar holoprosencephaly.

Prognosis depends on the form of holoprosencephaly. The severe forms are incompatible with prolonged survival. In the lobar type, the prognosis is less well defined, but mental retardation, olfactory and visual anomalies are often present Termination of pregnancy can be offered for the severe cases holoprosencephaly (semi-lobar, alobar).

6. Hydranencephaly

Hydranencephaly is characterized by the absence of the cerebral hemispheres, an incomplete or absent falx and a huge saclike structure containing cerebral spinal fluid covered by leptomeninges and dura. The brain stem is usually present, although the basal ganglia and cerebellum may be smaller than normal. The presence of the falx and of the cranial nerves demonstrates that the hemispheres have developed but have subsequently been destroyed (Dixon, 2005).

Etiology of this disorder includes: bilateral occlusion of the internal carotid or middle cerebral arteries, necrotizing vasculitis caused by infection (congenital cytomegalovirus, toxoplasmosis and herpes simplex infections), diffuse hypoxic-ischemic brain necrosis based on fetal hypoxia, leukomalacia formed by confluence of multiple cystic cavities and thromboplastic material from a deceased co-twin. The most accepted hypothesis to explain this particular lesion is interruption of the blood supply in early pregnancy (Barkovich, 2005). The occlusion of internal carotid arteries results in ischemic insult of the areas supplied by anterior and middle cerebral artery. There is variability in the extent of destruction of the cerebral hemispheres. Destruction may be complete or may spare portions of the temporal and occipital cortex. Liquefaction of the brain tissue in the area involved (usually the hemispheres), with replacement of the neural tissue by CSF and preservation of the membranes. Blood supply for the posterior brain fossa stays intact which explains the presence of brainstem and cerebellum

Hydranencephaly is a rare destructive brain lesions with prevalence to 0.1-0.2 in 1000 newborns. Hydranencephaly is found in 0.2% of infant autopsies. Recurrence risk is unknown. Aside from consequential arthrogryposis, hydranencephaly has been associated with syndromes including renal aplastic dysplasia, polyvalvular developmental heart defect, porencephaly, microcephaly and with trisomy 13 (Bendon *et al,* 1987). Familial cases are rare.

On ultrasound, hydrancephaly presents as a large cystic mass filling the entire cranial cavity with absence or discontinuity of the cerebral cortex (Figure 12.). Falx cerebri is partially missing or absent and brainstem is preserved. The pused and continuous color Doppler US show abnormal pathway and occlusion of the anterior cerebral artery crawling under the skull (Bernard *et al,* 2002; Stevenson *et al,* 2001).

The most common diagnostic problem is differentiation among hydranencephaly, extreme hydrocephalus, alobar holoprosencephaly and porencephaly. With extreme hydrocephaly, alobar holoprosencephaly or porencephaly, these structures should still be surrounded by a rim of cortex, and the choroid plexuses should be normally visible. Magnetic resonance imaging (MRI) and evoked potentials may serve as an additional means for confirming the ultrasound diagnosis (Hanigan & Aldrich, 1988). Diagnosis can be done prenatally by ultrasound (Lam & Tang, 2000).

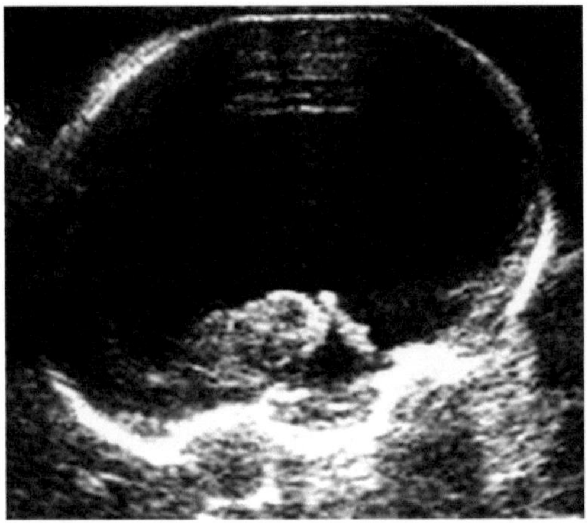

Fig. 12. Sagittal scan show sthe typical features of hydranencephaly.

The prognosis is universally very poor and incompatible with post-natal life. Hydranencephaly is associated with severe psychomotor delay, nystagmus, optic atrophy, epilepsy, and hypothermia. Survival may last several months if an intact hypothalamus permits thermoregulation, but most die in the first two years of life. It has been suggested termination of pregnancy when an antenatal diagnosis of hydranencephaly is made.

7. Schizencephaly

Schizencephaly is an uncommon CNS congenital disorder of neuronal migration, characterized abnormal cleft by brain (Oh *et al,* 2005). The cleft can be localized anywhere on the brain, but they are usually localized on the perisylvian regions. The cleft can be unilateral or bilateral and be either symmetric or asymmetric. The clefts may extend through the entire hemisphere from the ependymal lining of the lateral ventricles to the pial surface covering the cortex of some part of the brain. The gray matter lining can be dysplastic. There are two types of schizencephaly:

Type I: The clefts can be unilateral or bilateral and may be closed (fused lips). In closed-lip, the cleft walls are in apposition, causing obliteration of the CSF space within the cleft.

Type II: The clefts can be unilateral or bilateral and may be separated (open lips). In open-lips, the clefts walls are separated. The CSF fills the cleft from the lateral ventricles to the subarachnoid space that surrounds the hemispheres. The ventricle system may be enlarged, particularly with the open lip form of schizencephaly.

Schizencephaly has an extremely rare prevalence, with an unknown incidence. There is neither sex nor race predilection. Schizencephaly type II is more frequent than schizencephaly type I. Different CNS anomalies can be associated with schizencephaly: gray-matter heterotopias, polymicrogyria, arachnoid cysts, microcephaly, agenesis of the corpus callosus (Briellmann *et al,* 1998; Hayashi *et al,* 2002). The septum pellucidum is absent in 50-85 % of the patients and may coexist with septo-optic dysplasia. Some individuals affected by schizencephaly, may have an excessive accumulation of CSF in the brain and caused ventriculomegaly and the hydrocephaly with macrocrania.

Etiology of schizencephaly remains unclear, some environmental events have been proposed. No specific prenatal events have been identified, but genetic, toxic, metabolic, vascular of infectious etiology (congenital cytomegalovirus infection) can be responsible (Montenegro *et al,* 2002; Iannetti *et al,* 1998). Schizencephaly have an autosomal dominant inheritance with incomplete penetrance and variable expression. Familial cases have been reported, suggesting a possible genetic origin within a group of neuronal migration disorders (Guerrini & Carrozzo, 2001). Recent studies have linked schizencephaly with a mutated gene called EMX2 homeobox gene (Guerrini & Carrozzo, 2001; Granata et al, 1997). If the gene EMX-2 is missing or defective, nerve cell growth and migration will not occur normally and lead to the formation of the clefts associated with schizencephaly.

Two theories are currently accepted. One argues a failure in neuronal migration from the germinal matrix, while the other argues a post-migrational vascular insult (Montenegro *et al,* 2002; Oh *et al,* 2005). Schizencephaly results from an early, focal destruction of the germinal matrix and surrounding brain, before the hemispheres are fully formed. Schizencephaly can occur due to an abnormal neuronal migration from the germinal matrix zone. According to other authors, schizencephaly and polymicrogyria are the result of the same cortical damage, because of the frequent association of an unlayered cortex lining surrounding the cleft. Schizencephaly would be an extreme variant of cortical dysplasia in which the infolding of the cortex extends all the way into the lateral ventricles.

Schizencephaly may be suspected by the appearance of focal ventricular dilatation and by visualization of gray matter lined cleft on ultrasound (Hayashi *et al,* 2002). This space is filled with CSF. In unilateral schizencephaly, the clefts is only on one side of the brain, while in bilateral schizencephaly is on both sides (Figure 13.). The septum pellucidum is absent in most patient with schizencephaly. MRI is the best method to differentiate schizencephaly from porencephaly and arachnoid cyst (Hayashi *et al,* 2002; Liang *et al,* 2002).

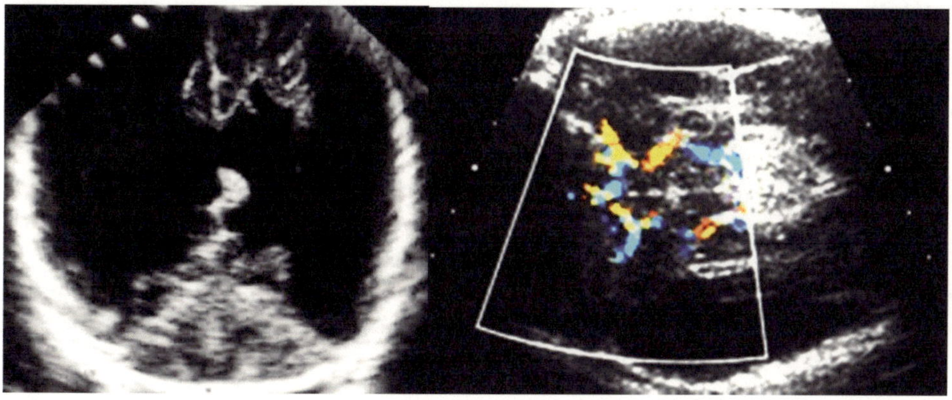

a b

Fig. 13. Coronal scan (A) and axial scan (B) show the typical features of bilateral schizencephaly.

The clinical features of schizencephaly are extremely variable. Usually the severity of these symptoms is related to the extent of cortex involved in the defect and associated CNS anomalies (Denis *at al* 2000; Hayashi *et al,* 2002). Children with unilateral clefts have often hemiparesis, but may also have mild-to-moderate developmental delay. Children with bilateral clefts have severe mental and motor impairments, early onset of epilepsy and frequently blindness, deafness. Sometimes, closed-lip schizencephaly may not present clinically until later during the childhood and may live to early adulthood.

8. Lissencephaly

Cerebral cortical development is an extremely complex process, comprising three major, but overlapping, steps: cell proliferation, neuronal migration and cortical organization. Neuronal migration disorders (also, and better, called cortical developmental anomaly) are caused by abnormal proliferation, migration, and organization (lamination, gyration, and sulcation). Lissencephaly is a rare cortical developmental disorder, with reduced or absent brain gyri, which is caused by abnormal neuronal migration in the neocortex.

The incidence lissencephaly is unknown but rare. There is female predilection. Lissencephaly have been associated with deletion of a number of genes on chromosome 17p13, including *LIS1*. Identification of *LIS1* as the causative gene for lissencephaly did not come until 1993, and the role of *DCX* in both lissencephaly and subcortical band heterotopia was not determined until 1998. *DCX* is located on the long arm of the X chromosome and therefore is inherited in an X-linked dominant form, with female subjects showing a milder phenotype (subcortical band heterotopia) than male subjects (anterior greater than posterior lissencephaly). If de novo deletion or translocation occurs, the recurrence risk is low. If the translocation is inherited from one parent (who has a balanced translocation), the recurrence risk may be as high as 25%.

Lissencephaly is characterized by agyria, accompanied or not by pachygyria, minimal or no ventriculomegaly, and characteristic dysmorphic features (Verloes *et al*, 2007). The most frequently associated anomalies are duodenal atresia, urinary tract abnormalities, congenital heart defects, cryptorchidism, inguinal hernia, clinodactyly, polydactyly, and ear anomalies may be found. The classification of lissencephaly has undergone significant revision in the last decade, as a result of recent discoveries regarding the molecular biological basis of such malformations, and findings on MRI and autopsy. There are three main groups of lissencephaly (Barkovich *et al*, 2001).

Group A lissencephaly (or classical lissencephaly) is characterized by agyria with or without pachygyria, a wide cortical mantle and minimal or no hydrocephalus. In classical lissencephaly (agyria/pachygyria), the normal six-layered cortex is replaced by an abnormally thick four-layered cortex and characterized by simplified or absent gyration. The incidence of all forms of type I lissencephaly is around 1 in 100,000 births. The subtypes of group A lissencephaly are:

1. Miller-Dieker syndrome is associated with a deletion at the chromosome 17p13.3 locus. This syndrome has lissencephaly combined with dysmorphic facial features and other possible associated CNS anomalies (dysgenesis of the corpus callosum, ventriculomegaly, midline calcifications, and mild cortical cerebellar dysplasia). Microcephaly is common. Associated abnormalities include heart malformations, omphalocele, kidney dysplasia, and genital anomalies). Transverse palmar creases and clinodactyly are common. Among extracranial abnormalities, the most common is intrauterine growth restriction.

2. In Norman-Roberts syndrome, no abnormal karyotype is fond. This syndrome is autosomal recessively inherited. It is a type I lissencephaly with sloping forehead and other minor facial features described in a consanguineous family.

3. Isolated *type I* lissencephaly is not associated with deletion at the chromosome 17p13.3 locus or abnormalities limited to the *LIS1* gene. Patients with isolated lissencephaly do not have other congenital anomalies or severe dysmorphic features.

Group B lissencephaly (or type II) is characterised by global disorganisation of cerebral organogenesis with an uneven cortical surface Lissencephaly, type II typically has hydrocephalus and additional serious CNS defects. The subtypes of group B lissencephaly are:

1. HARD+/-E syndrome, an acronym for Hydrocephalus, Agyria, Retinal dysplasia, Encephalocele (Walker-Warburg syndrome), is an autosomal recessive lethal disorder. Associated abnormalities include other serious CNS malformations such as dysgenesis of the corpus callosum, cerebellar dysplasia with Dandy-Walker malformation, and white brain substance atrophy are found.

2. Cerebro-oculomuscular syndrome with congenital muscular dysplasia is possibly a variant of the HARD+/-E syndrome, and is supposed to be autosomal recessively inherited. Other subtypes of type II lissencephaly are possible.

Group C lissencephaly is found in lissencephaly associated with Neu-Laxova syndrome which is a lethal autosomal recessive inherited disorder consisting of growth retardation, microcephaly, lissencephaly, dysgenesis of the corpus callosum, intracranial calcifications, cerebellar hypoplasia, facial dysmorphism, microphthalmia, exophthalmus, cataracts, absent eyelids, hydrops, ichthyosis, contractures of extremities and syndactyly.

Lssencephaly may be suspected if appear a smooth gyral pattern, ventriculomegaly, and a prominent subarachnoid space on ultrasound (Barkovich *et al,* 2001) (Figure 14.). The progressive microcephaly and failure of development of both sulci and gyri (which in normal conditions is well defined from 26 to 28 weeks) are suggestive of lissencephaly (Fong *et al,* 2004). MRI may be better able to detect the pachygyric appearance of the cerebral cortex and subcortical band heterotopia (Garel et al, 2001; Levente, 2005).

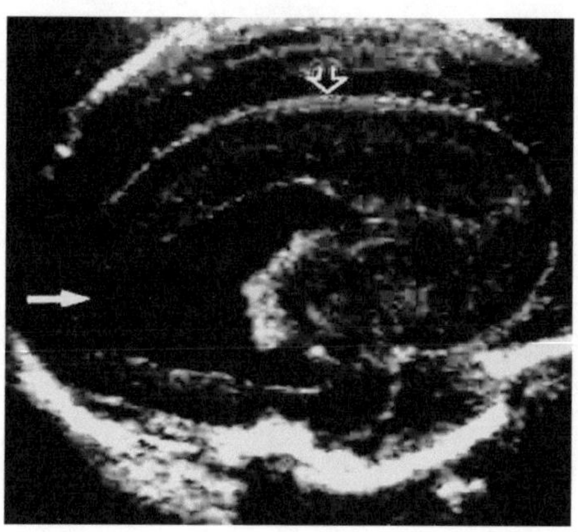

Fig. 14. Coronal scan shows the typical features of lissencephaly.

The prognosis of lissencephaly is universally poor, regardless of etiological type, and death occurs usually within the first 2 years of life. Usually severe mental retardation affects these patients. Failure to thrive, infantile spasms, and seizures are also expected.

9. Porencephaly

The term 'porencephaly' includes every type of destructive brain lesion with cavitary character, i.e. a fluid-filled spaces within the brain that commonly communicates with the ventricles, subarachnoid spaces, or both. It involves the destruction of previously developed brain tissue, with subsequent cavity formation. It may be isolated or associated with ventriculomegaly. Some authors consider two types of porencephaly.

Type I porencephaly or encephaloclastic porencephaly is due to parenchymal damage followed by liquification/reabsorption, resulting from an insult (ischemia, hemorrhage, etc.) during the 3rd trimester. It is more frequent and usually unilateral. It has a round or irregular shape.

Type II porencephaly or schizencephalic porencephaly, which is usually bilateral, caused by abnormal neural migration and cortical organization. It is best considered separately as a primary developmental abnormality.

Etiology of porencephaly disorder includes: ischemic episode, trauma, demise of one twin, intercerebral hemorrhage and infection (Scher *et al,* 1991). This occurs when the immature brain has a propensity to dissolution and cavitations (due to high water content or a deficient astroglial response). The timing of ischemic injury (maybe as early as the 2nd trimester) is closely related to porencephaly and hydranencephaly.

Porencephaly is a rare destructive brain lesion with prevalence to 0.1-0.2 in 1000 newborns. Risk of non-chromosomal syndromes is low. Type II porencephaly may be associated with orofaciodigital syndrome type I, and other CNS anomalies. The most frequently associated anomalies are hydrocephalus.

On ultrasound, porencephaly appears as a unilateral cystic lesion, usually communicating with the ipsilateral ventricle and/or the subarachnoid space (Figure 15.). A porencephalic cyst never causes a mass effect, which is observed with arachnoid cysts and other cystic

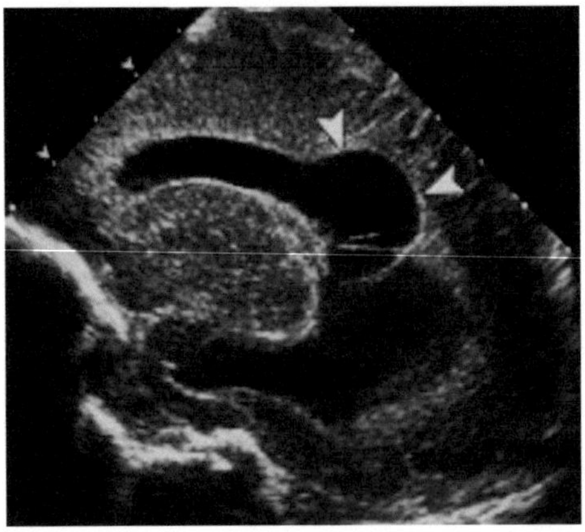

Fig. 15. Sagittal scan shows the typical features of porencephalic cyst.

mass lesions. This condition is an acquired brain insult and should be differentiated from schizencephaly of migration disorder. The cystic walls and the content of the cyst may vary according to the gestational age at which the insult occurs. If it is secondary to hemorrhage, it is possible to visualize a hyperechoic focus evolving into an anechoic CSF-filled cyst. Diagnosis can be done prenatally by ultrasound (Meizner & Elchalal, 1996).

Prognosis is variable, depending on the timing and extent of the lesion. Epilepsy psychomotor retardation and cerebral palsy often occur. In type II, due to the bilaterality of the lesion and the tendency to be part of a syndrome, the prognosis is worse. A ventriculoperitoneal shunt should be applied if hydrocephalus progresses.

10. Arachnoid cysts

Arachnoid cysts are congenital lesions of the arachnoid membrane that expand with CSF secretion. They exist between the brain substance and dura and that may exist separately as a loculated accumulation between two arachnoid membranes or may communicate with the subarachnoid space. They represent 1% of all intracranial masses in newborns and they are found at 0.5% of autopsies. Arachnoid cysts are fluid-filled cavities lined completely or partially by the arachnoid membrane. The cysts are mostly single, but two or more can occasionally be observed. Arachnoid cysts have been found anywhere in the CNS, including the spinal canal. The most frequent locations are the surface of the cerebral hemispheres in the sites of the major fissures (sylvian, rolandic, and interhemispheric), the region of sella turcica, the anterior fossa, and the middle fossa (Nakamura *et al*, 2001). Less frequently, they are seen in the posterior fossa. Arachnoid cysts may increase or decrease in size.

Arachnoid cysts have been associated with hydrocephalus, Aicardi syndrome, glutaric acid-uria type I, and unbalanced X,9 translocation. Interhemispheric cysts are often associated with dysgenesis of the corpus callosum (Hirohata *et al*, 1992). Recurrence risk is unknown.

Intracranial arachnoid cysts may be primary (congenital) or secondary (acquired). Congenital types are believed to be formed by maldevelopment arachnoid membranes and do not freely communicate with subarachnoid space. Acquired types are formed as the result of hemorrhage, trauma, and infection and often communicate with subarachnoid space. Arachnoid cysts have the potential to grow as the result of some communication with the subarachnoid space. The accumulation of fluid is believed to result from a ball valve mechanism. Furthermore, a choroid plexus-like tissue within the cyst wall, which secretes CSF and thus contributes to a progressive distension of the lesion, has been reported by several investigators. It contains clear cerebrospinal fluid and has been diagnosed prenatally by ultrasound.

On ultrasound, arachnoid cysts present as a well-defined anechoic cystic structure with adjacent mass effect. The primary manifestation of an arachnoid cyst is a localized fluid collection occasionally causing hydrocephallus. Large arachnoid cysts may obstruct the circulation of CSF, leading to secondary obstructive hydrocephalus. The cyst can obstruct the foramen of Monro, displace the aqueduct posteriorly, and block the basal cisterns. Application of color Doppler will not demonstrate high flow (Figure 16.).

The differential diagnosis from other cystic lesions may be difficult. Porencephaly is often associated with ventriculomegaly, communicates with the ventricles and follows a vascular distribution. Brain tumors are usually solid or of mixed echogenicity and are rarely completely cystic. Posterior fossa arachnoid cysts should be differentiated from Dandy-Walker malformation. The main criterion in these cases is the integrity of the cerebellar vermis in arachnoid cysts. Suprasellar arachnoid cysts are rounded and should be differentiated from a large third ventricle. The dilated third ventricle appears oval with tapered edges posteriorly when aqueductal stenosis is present. An arachnoid cyst in the midline should be differentiated from dysgenesis of corpus callosum with an associated interhemispheric cyst. In cases of corpus callosal dysgenesis, the enlarged third ventricle is high in location at the level of the lateral ventricles, and the ventricular atria are prominent. A vein of Galen aneurysm, is a midline occipital lesion with characteristic Doppler flow.

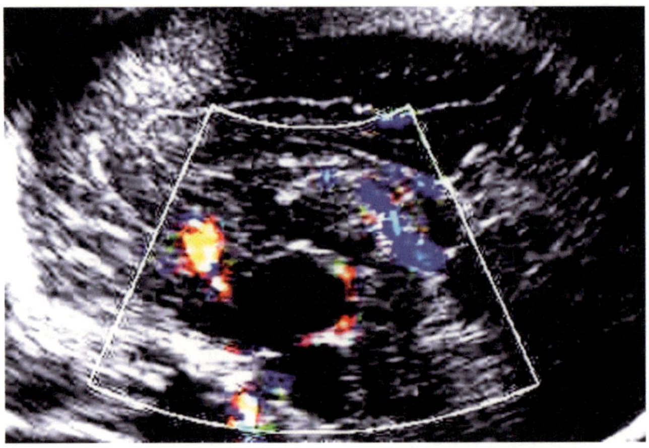

Fig. 16. Sagittal scan shows the typical features of arachnoid cysts.

Prognosis is generally good (Elbers & Furness, 1999). In many cases, arachnoid cysts are asymptomatic, but they may cause epilepsy, mild motor or sensory abnormalities, or hydrocephalus. Depending on the location and extent of the lesion, these cysts can be resected or shunted. Conversely, suprasellar arachnoid cysts are rare, representing approximately 10% of intracranial arachnoid cysts, however, they have a propensity to become symptomatic and they may manifest with hydrocephalus, visual impairment, and endocrine dysfunctions (typically precocious puberty).

11. Posterior fossa cystic lesions

Despite decades of knowledge of the existence of posterior fossa cystic anomalies and efforts to understand their pathogenesis, there is little consensus about how these malformations occur and how they cause clinical symptoms/signs (Altman, 1992; Barkovich *et al,* 1989).

However, their differential diagnosis can be particularly difficult because the recognition of the subtle anatomic features that differentiate them may be challenging or sometimes impossible.

Some cysts are related to massive dilatation of the fourth ventricle, others to persistence of embryonic structures, such as Blake's pouch, others to malformative dilatation of subarachnoid spaces, and others to true arachnoid loculations.

The mainstay of the diagnosis is represented by the assessment of a number of direct and indirect signs, including the following: the relationship of the cyst with the fourth ventricle and subarachnoid spaces; the morphology, position and biometry of the vermis and the cerebellar hemispheres, association with hydrocephalus; the size of the posterior fossa and the position of the tentorium.

11.1 Mega cisterna magna

The cisterna magna is the basal cistern behind and below the cerebellum. Mega cisterna magna is defined as a cystic posterior fossa malformation characterized by an intact vermis, an enlarged cisterna magna, freely communicating with the perimedullary subarachnoid spaces, absence of hydrocephalus, and a normal size of the fourth ventricle. The tentorium cerebelli is superiorly displaced in almost 10% of cases.

Mega cisterna magna occurs in approximately 1% of all brains imaged postnatally. Mega cisterna magna has been associated with infarction, inflammation, and infection, particularly cytomegalovirus, as well as with chromosomal abnormalities, especially trisomy 18. In the absence of other findings to suggest a posterior fossa lesion, a mega cisterna magna is unlikely to be clinically significant.

On ultrasound, normal cisterna magna characteristically measures 3-8 mm when measurements are taken in the midsagittal plane from the posterior lip of the foramen magnum to the caudal margin of the inferior vermis (Goodwin & Quisling, 1983). Ultrasound examination reveals a cystic posterior fossa malformation characterized by an intact vermis, an enlarged cisterna magna, absence of hydrocephalus, and a normal size of the fourth ventricle (Figure 17.). The extent of the CSF collection is variable; it may remain purely infravermian or it may extend far beyond the normal borders of the cisterna magna laterally, posteriorly, and superiorly, reaching in some cases the quadrigeminal plate cistern. The tentorium are usually in normal position.

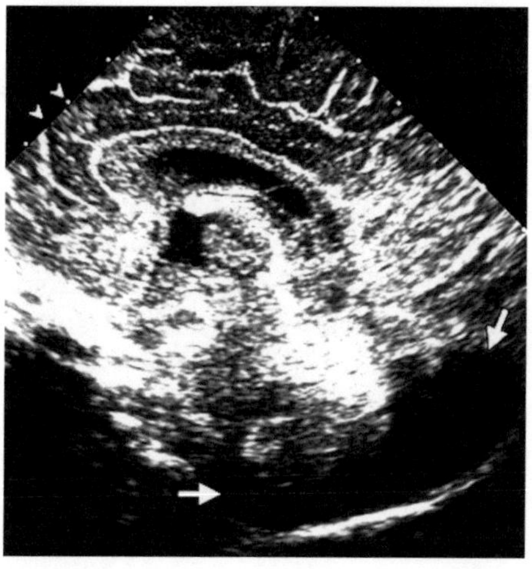

Fig. 17. Sagittal scan shows the typical features of Mega cisterna magna.

Prognosis is commonly favorable if Mega cisterna magna is isolated. In syndromic conditions, the final prognosis is that of the underlying syndrome.

11.2 Blake's pouch cyst

The Blake's pouch is a normal, transient embryological structure (superior medullary velum), which initially does not communicate with the surrounding sub-arachnoid spaces. Subsequent spontaneous perforation of the pouch forms the foramen of Magendie. If the Blake's pouch fails to perforate, CSF accumulates and determines the fingerlike expansion Blake's pouch cyst within the posterior fossa and produce hydrocephalus.

Some authors put forward the theory that Blake's pouch cyst and retrocerebellar arachnoid cysts are the same entity because at some stage the communication with the fourth ventricle is lost and contact with the developing arachnoid matter is made (Strand *et al,* 1993). Another authors clearly distinguish between Blake's pouch cysts and retrocerebellar arachnoid cysts although they recognize differentiation of the two on imaging is difficult and can only be resolved on histological analysis (Calabro *et al,* 2000).

Sonographically, Blake's pouch cysts is characterized by a normal but displaced cerebellar vermis, a CSF collection in the posterior fossa, consisting of the expanded and imperforated Blake's pouch widely communicating with the fourth ventricle. Ventriculomegaly/ hydrocephalus is often associated. The tentorium is usually in normal position. A normal appearance of the cerebellar vermis rules out the diagnosis of the Dandy-Walker malformation, in which the vermis is agnetic/hypoplastic and rotated counterclockwise (Calabro *et al,* 2000).

The prognosis of Blake's pouch cysts is generally good.

11.3 Dandy-Walker malformation

The term Dandy-Walker malformation was suggested to describe a malformation consisting of a cystic enlargement of the fourth ventricle associated with partial or complete agenesis of the vermis (Nelson *et al,* 2004)

Incidence of the Dandy-Walker is about 1 in 25,000–35,000 births.

There is a high association with other CNS abnormalities (in 50–60% of cases), including failed commissuration, cortical formation malformations, midline anomalies and encephalocoeles. An association with facial clefts and other extra-CNS anomalies (especially congenital heart disease and urinary anomalies) has been described, often in the context of chromosomal and genetic syndromes. Risk of chromosomal anomalies is high, with up to 35% of cases being associated with aneuploidy, mainly trisomies 18 and 13. The most common syndromes that can be associated with the Dandy-Walker malformation are: Walker-Warburg syndrome, Meckel-Gruber syndrome, Aicardi syndrome and Neu-Laxova syndrome.

The Dandy-Walker malformation is a result of defective development of the structures originating from the rhomboencephalic roof (Calabro *et al,* 2000; Nelson *et al,* 2004). Failure of assimilation of the area membranacea anterior, leading to anomalous development of the fourth ventricle, atresia of the foramen of Magendie and sometimes the foramen of Luschka. The cystic dilatation of the fourth ventricle fills the posterior fossa and extends into cisterna magna, which is compressed between the dilated fourth ventricle and the dura mater. Ventriculomegaly develops in up to 80% of cases. The high insertion of the tentorium encountered in the Dandy-Walker malformation is considered an indicator that the malformation occurred before the end of the embryonic period.

On ultrasound, the Dandy–Walker malformation is characterized by an expansion of the posterior cranial fossa with upward displacement of the tentorium, a cystic dilatation of the fourth ventricle, and partial or complete vermian agenesis (Figure 18.). In addition, when present, the cerebellar vermis is rotated counter clockwise. Some cases of Dandy–Walker malformation show a partial agenesis/ hypoplasia, whereas others feature vermian dysplasia.

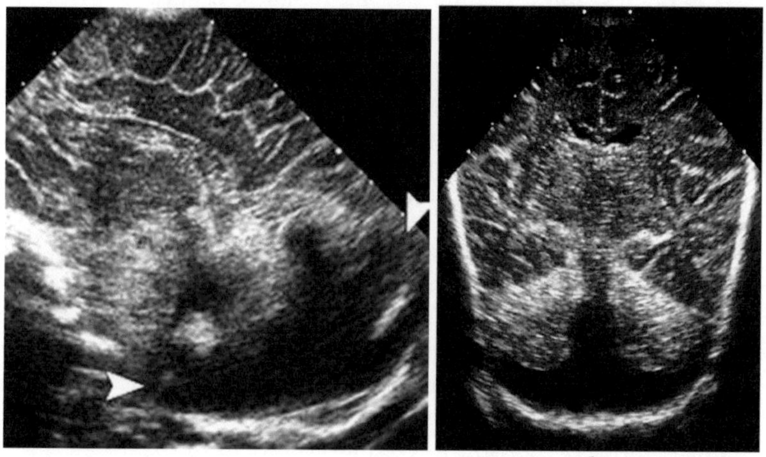

a b

Fig. 18. Sagittal scan (A) and coronal (B)show the typical features of Dandy–Walker malformation.

Prognosis is poor when associated with other CNS anomalies and chromosomal and genetic syndromes (Klein *et al,* 2004). Isolated the Dandy–Walker malformation forms have a better intellectual prognosis and lower mortality

Less-pronounced malformations are often termed Dandy-Walker varianta.

The Dandy–Walker variant has a very similar appearance but there is a lesser degree of hypoplasia of the cerebellar vermis. The foramen of Magendie is, however, patent. The fourth ventricle is less dilated. The Dandy–Walker variant is a mild form of the Dandy-Walker malformation or represents a generalized form of cerebellar hypoplasia. However, the demarcation between classic Dandy-Walker malformation and Dandy-Walker variant is vague, and thus the term Dandy-Walker continuum is more appropriate. To further simplify these lesions, the definition of Dandy-Walker malformation has been modified and Blake's pouch cyst has been included in the "Dandy-Walker continuum".

12. Vein of Galen aneurysm

The vein of Galen is part off the venous sinus complex which drains blood from brain. Aneurysm of the vein of Galen is a complex arteriovenous malformation consisting of multiple communications between the system of the vein of Galen and the cerebral arteries (carotid and/or vertebrobasiliar systems). These vessels are located in the brain deeply and posteriorly above the pineal gland, in the subarachnoid space called "cistern of the great cerebral vein of Galen". There three types described: arteriovenous fistula, arteriovenous malformation with ectasia of the vein of Galen and varix of the vein of Galen (Raybaud *et al,* 1989). The vein of Galen malformation is a form of embryonic arteriovenous shunt. Other venous anomalies, such as anomalous dural sinuses and sinus stenosis, are commonly present in association with vein of Galen malformation.

Incidence of aneurysm the vein of Galen is rare. It represents 1% of all vascular brain malformations. It is more common in males than females. It is often associated with other more extensive cerebral abnormalities. It may be associated with secondary hydrocephalus due to compression of the aqueduct and with high-output heart failure and non-immune hydrops due to the arteriovenous fistula (Brunelle, 1997). Severe high-output cardiac failure is caused by a marked increase of cardiac preload from venous return of the brain due to the 'steal' phenomenon. The 'steal' phenomenon, with diversion of blood from the parenchyma to the aneurysm, may further result in brain infarcts and periventricular white matter lesions.

Ultrasound examination reveals a large echo-free supratentorial cystic structure with high velocity flow on Doppler examination (Figure 19.). This lies posterior to the third ventricle, and may extend asymmetrically across the midline. Size of this cystic structure depends on volume of shunt. The sagittal sinus is reported as dilated in most cases. The feeding arteries are difficult to analyze, but a tortuous network of dilated arteries is usually visible in the region of the malformation. Demonstration of blood flow in the cystic structure enables the diagnosis of an aneurysm of the vein of Galen to be made, as opposed to that of an abnormality of other intracranial midline structures, for example arachnoid or porencephalic cyst, Dandy-Walker malformation or intracerebral hematoma. However, when a clot has formed, it may be iso-or even hyperechoic (Vijayarghavan *et al,* 2006).

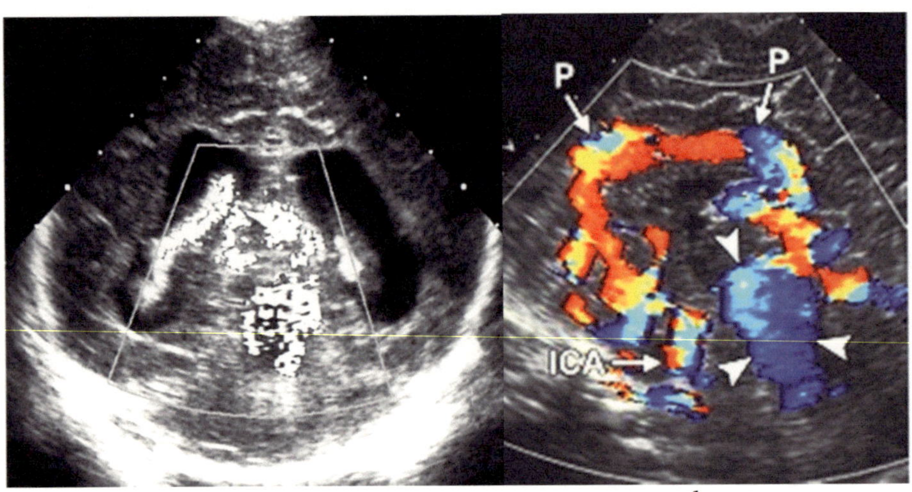

a b

Fig. 19. Coronal scan (A) and sagittal scan (B) show the typical features of the vein of Galen malformation.

Prognosis of aneurysm the vein of Galen is poor when cardiac failure and hydrops is present. Risk of intrauterine or early neonatal death due to congestive heart failure, requires agressive postnatal care. Although the vein of Galen aneurysms may become symptomatic in the elderly, they are more typically diagnosed in the neonatal period. The common clinical features in the neonate are cardiomegaly with congestive heart failure and increased intracranial pressure with hydrocephaly or cranial bruit. Focal neurological deficit, seizures and hemorrhages are less common findings. If possible, method of treatment is emergency embolization or surgery. However, there are some reports of spontaneous thrombosis and calcification of aneurysm of the vein of Galen (Nikas *et al*, 1999; Chapman & Hockley, 1989).

13. Neural tube defects

Neural tube defects are the most frequent CNS malformations and amount to about 1-2 cases per 1000 births. There have been many reported remarkable reductions in the prevalence of neural tube defects after the use of folic acid supplementation and fortification, although some have reported no decline in the anencephaly rate. Neural tube defects includes different anomalies deriving from failed closure of the neural tube between the 3rd and the 4th week of development, the best known being anencephaly, cefalocele, and spina bifida.

13.1 Anencephaly

Anencephaly results from failure of anterior neural tube closure and occurs before 24 days of gestation. Anencephaly is a lethal anomaly characterized by the absence of cerebral hemispheres and cranial vault. Most of the cranial vault is absent. It is the most common CNS malformation. Its incidence is 0.1 in 1000 births. In neonates, the anomaly is more frequent in females than in males. The incidence of anencephaly in abortion material has been found to be five times greater than that observed at birth. The risk of recurrence of anencephaly is 5% to 13%. Anencephaly is associated with myelomeningocele, microcephaly and amniotic band syndrome. Extra-cranial abnormalities occur in some cases and included omphaloceles and clubfoot.

Anencephaly has a multifactorial etiology. Genetic factors seem important because of familial incidence, whereas geographic variation suggests an environmental cause. An increased incidence of anencephaly and other neural tube defects occur in women who have diabetes during pregnancy. Also, women who take valproic acid for a seizure disorder are at increased risk for anencephaly if their medication has been consumed prior to conception or during the first trimester of pregnancy. The most widely accepted theory is that in most cases, because of a failure of development of the cranial vault bones, the encephalic structures, covered only by the meninges, are in time subject to extensive destruction, with consequent transformation of the encephalon into a mass of soft tissue adhering to the base of the cranium (cerebral-vascular area).

On ultrasound, the anencephalic foetus have a typical froglike appearance (bulging eyes, cleft lip or palate, a large tongue, and a very short neck) (Chatzipapas & Whitlow, 1999). This anomaly is incompatible with life. Approximately 75% of these neonates are stillborn, and the remainder die within the first hours or days of life. Anencephalic infants are a potential source of organs for transplantation (Trugg & Fletcher, 1989).

13.2 Cephalocele

Cephalocele is usually considered to be a restricted disorder of anterior neural tube closure. It occurs before 26 days of gestation. Cephalocele is characterized by protrusion of intracranial structures through a cranial bone defect. The herniated anatomic structures can consist of meninges only (meningocephalocele) or meninges plus cerebral tissue (encephalomeningocele). Cephaloceles are defined anatomically according to their location (frontal, parietal, occipital, frontoethmoidal, etc.). Neural tissue (most often from the occipital lobe) in the encephalocele usually displays a normal gyration and underlying white matter and is connected to the brain through a narrow neck. The most common location is occipital in Europe and the USA, although frontal cephaloceles are more frequent in South-East Asia.

This is relatively high percent (14–18%) of chromosomal anomalies (e.g., trisomy 13 and 18). The syndromes possibly associated with cephalocele are Meckel-Gruber syndrome, amniotic band syndrome, frontonasal dysplasia and Walker-Warburg syndrome. Associated anomalies occur in up to 70–80% of cases and included agenesis of the corpus callosum, ventriculomegaly, holoprosencephaly, spina bifida and microcephaly. Among extracerebral anomalies, the most frequently associated are cardiac anomalies and skeletal dysplasias.

According to the most widely accepted theory, cephalocele is caused by a lack of fusion of the neural tube in its specific closing sites, although some authors claim that postneurulation events with anomalies of the mesenchymal induction phases of the nervous tissue are responsible for the lesion.

Ultrasound diagnosis is based on the recognition of a cystic (meningocephalocele) or complex (meningoencephalocele) formation of variable size protruding through a skull defect, often localized in the occipital region (Figure 20.). In cases where the cephalocele is located in the lower occipital region or upper cervical area, cerebellum is usually present in the encephalocele and often associated with type III Chiari malformation. Chiari III malformation is a high cervical encephalomeningocele in which the medulla, fourth ventricle, and virtually the entire cerebellum reside.

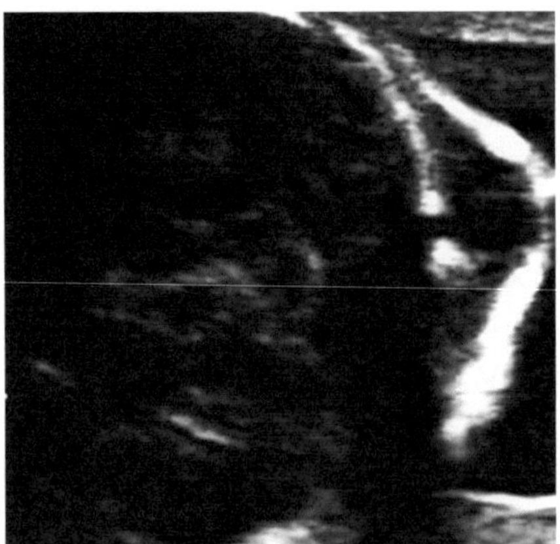

Fig. 20. Axial scan shows the typical features of occipital cephalocele.

Prognosis is depending on the dimensions and the location of the lesion, on the presence of cerebral tissue in the herniated sack, and on any association with hydrocephaly or microcephaly or other extracranial anomalies. The postnatal mortality rate varies from 30% to 50%, depending on the above-mentioned parameters. Very large lesions have an unfavorable prognosis, while small cephaloceles can be corrected surgically.

13.3 Spina bifida

The term 'spina bifida' is still commonly used as a synonym for spinal dysraphism, although it properly refers to defective fusion of posterior spinal bony elements. The terms spina bifida aperta or cystica and spina bifida occulta were once used to refer to open spinal dysraphism and closed spinal dysraphism, respectively but have been progressively discarded. Spina bifida encompasses a broad spectrum of abnormalities. Lesions are commonly subdivides into ventral and dorsal defects. Ventral defects are extremely rare and are characterized by the splitting of the vertebral body and the occurrence of a cyst that is neuroenteric in origin. This lesion is generally seen in the lower cervical or upper thoracic vertebrae. Dorsal defects are the most common. Closed spinal dysraphisms represents approximately 15% of the cases and is characterized by a small defect completely covered by skin. Closed spinal dysraphisms are considered to be disorders of caudal neural tube formation (secondary neurulation) and include distortion of the spinal cord or roots by fibrous bands and adhesions, intraspinal lipomas, epidermoid cysts, fibrolipomas, tethered cord (the most common condition), and diastematomyelia. In many cases, this condition is completely asymptomatic and is diagnosed only incidentally at radiographic examination of the spine. In other instances, there is an area of hypertrichosis, pigmented or dimpled skin, or the presence of subcutaneous lipomas. Closed spinal defects are extremely difficult to diagnose. Open spinal dysraphism is the most frequent lesion. The neural canal may be exposed, or the defect may be covered by a thin meningeal membrane. More often, the lesion appears as a cystic tumor (spina bifida cystica). If the tumor contains purely meninges, the lesion is referred to us a meningocele. More frequently, neural tissue is part of the mass, and the name myelomeningocele is used. The skin and muscles above the defect are absent. Approximately 75% of myelomeningoceles have a lumbar localization.

The incidence varies according to many factors, such as geographical area, ethnic differences, and seasonal variation. Spinal defects are more frequent in Caucasians than in Orientals or blacks. Spina bifida has a multifactorial etiology. The vast majority of cases are thought to be due to an interaction of genetic factors (chromosomal abnormalities and in single-gene disorders) with environmental factors (such as valproate exposure or maternal diabetes mellitus). Risk of chromosomal anomalies (trisomy 13, trisomy 18 and triploidy) is 8–16%. The syndromes possibly associated with spina bifida are Meckel syndrome, HARDE syndrome, Marfans syndrome and Ehlers–Danlos syndromes.

Cranial ultrasound should always be performed in neonates with spinal dysraphisms, as there may be associated a variety of intracranial abnormalities, including ventriculomegaly and hypoplasia of the posterior fossa structures. All infants with spina bifida have some degree of Arnold-Chiari type II malformation (D'Addario *et al*, 2001). Arnold-Chiari type II malformation is complex congenital anomaly of the hindbrain characterized by displacement of cerebellar tonsils, parts of the cerebellum, fourth ventricle, pons, and medulla oblongata through the foramen magnum into the spinal canal. In 95% of the cases it is accompanied by hydrocephalus and myelomeningocele. Clubfoot may develop in a significant percentage of cases. Neonates with lumbal spinal dysraphisms should have a hydronephrosis and renal ultrasound should also be perfomed.

A larger bone and cartilage-free portals may be present at the site of the lesion on a spinal ultrasonography. A meningocele contains only CSF and no neural elements (Figure 21.a). The sac is clearly cystic and occasionally communicates directly with the extra-axial space. Myelomeningocele may be unilocular or multi-locular sacs but always contain hyperechoic nerve roots. Ultrasonography should not be performed on open lesions. Both myelomeningoceles and meningoceles are associated with a tethered low-lying spinal cord and diastematomyelia or syringomyelia. Tethering of the spinal cord occurs in 70%–90% of these neonates. If spinal cord lies posteriorly and appears fixed then tethering should be suspected. In cases in which there is a low tethered cord, the conus is low and the spinal cord is displaced dorsally. There is lack of normal cord pulsatility, and the filum terminale is thickened to over 2 mm. The thickened filum terminale may be fibrous or lipomatous. Lipomas are highly echogenic and are easily identified on sonograms. Hydromyelia or syringomyelia occurs in 40-80% of these neonates. These conditions result from disturbance of cerebrospinal fluid circulation. Hydromyelia and syringomyelia always occur cranial to the placode and may be focal or involve the entire spinal cord and spinal US shows dilatation of the central canal of the spinal cord (Figure 21.b).

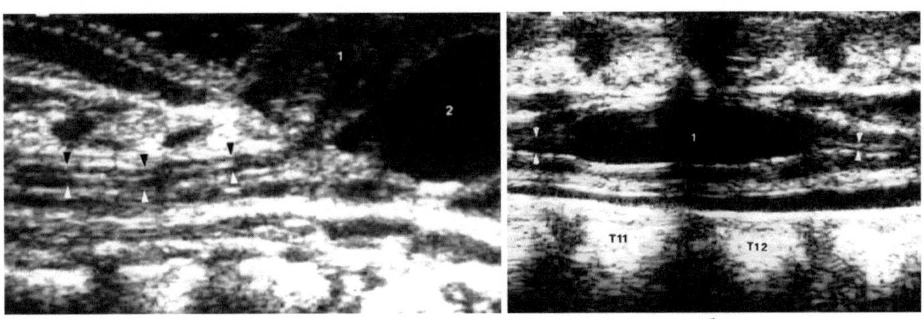

a b

Fig. 21. Longitudinal scan shows the typical features of meningocele (A) and syringomyelia (B).

There is high association with ventriculomegaly and Arnold-Chiari type II malformation. Ultrasound diagnosis of the Arnold-Chiari type II malformation is based on the recognition of: ventriculomegaly, banana sign (abnormal anterior curvature of the cerebellar hemispheres), caudal displacement of fastigium of fourth ventrcle and cerebellar hemispheres, obliteration of the cisterna magna (< 2 mm), and a hypoplastic cerebellar hemispheres (Figure 22.).

Spina bifida is a serious congenital anomaly. Prognosis depend on the location and extent of the lesion (cervical and high thoracic lesions are frequently fatal), kyphoscoliosis and other major structural abnormalities. The presence of severe hydrocephaly has always been considered a poor prognostic sign. The stillbirth rate is estimated as 25%. The untreated infants die within the first few months of life. Survival rate of those treated in the immediate neonatal period approaches 40% at seven years. Clinical symptoms are variable (absent, minimal, moderate, or severe) according to the degree of neural tissue involvement. Varying degree of paresis (often severe) of the legs and sphincter dysfunction are the major clinical signs. Intellectual and psychological disturbances are also frequently associated.

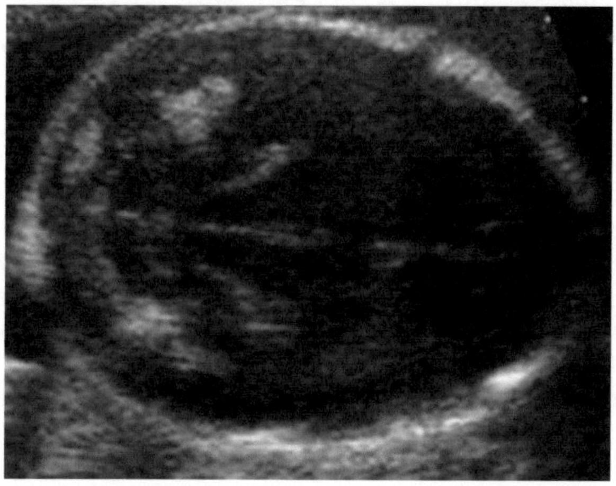

Fig. 22. Axial scan shows the tipical features of the Arnold-Chiari type II malformation.

14. Conclusions

Congenital brain anomalies are some of the most common of all congenital abnormalities These abnormalities are often evident of birth, but some brain malformations may not be immediately obvious. The neonates with dysmorphic features or abnormal neurologic behaviour may suggest cerebral malformation, and various imaging techniques are essential for fether clarification. In the neonatal period cranial US can be used as the initial modality to exclude a major structural malformation. Cranial US is non-invasive highly sensitive, safe, easily repeatable and cost effective for detecting congenital anomalies of the brain in both preterm and full-term neonates. It may provide important information regarding the anatomic location, size, and shape of congenital brain anomalies as well as their mass effect on adjacent structures. Cranial US are correlated with anatomical and pathological findings and clinical outcomes. Familiarity with the US features of congenital brain anomalies is therefore an extremely valuable tool, as it facilitates an accurate diagnosis and treatment when necessary.

15. References

Altman N, Naidich TP, Brafmann BH. (1992). Posterior fossa malformations. *AJNR*, Vol. 13, No. 2, (March 1992), pp. 691-724.

Atlas S, Shkolinik A, Naidich T. (1985). Sonographic recognition of agenesis of the corpus callosum. *AJR*, Vol. 145, No.1, (July 1985), pp. 167-173.

Barkovich AJ. (Ed).(2005). *Pediatric neuroimaging*. 4rd ed.Lippincott Williams & Wilkins Publishers, ISBN 0-7817-5766-5, New York, USA.

Barkovich AJ, Kjos BO, Norman D, Edwards MS. (1989). Revised classification of posterior fossa cyst and cystlike malformations based on the results of multiplanar MR imaging. *AJR*, Vol.153 , No.6, (December 1989), pp. 1289–1300.

Barkovich AJ, Kuzniecky RI, Jackson GD, Guerrini R, Dobyns WB. (2005). A developmental and genetic classification for malformations of cortical development. *Neurology*, Vol. 65, (December 2005), No. 12, pp. 1873-1887.

Barkovich AJ, Kuzniecky RI, Jackson GD, Guerrini R, Dobyns WB. (2001). Clasification system for malformations of cortical development update. *Neurology*, Vol. 57, No. 12, (December 2001), pp. 2168-2178.

Barkovich AJ. (1990). Apparent atypical callosal dysgenesis: analysis of MR findings and their relationship to holoprosencephaly. *AJNR*, Vol. 11, No. 2, (March 1990), pp. 333-339.

Barkovich A, Norman D. (1988) Anomalies of the corpus callosum: correlation with further anomalies of the brain. *AJR*, Vol. 151, No. 1, (July 1998), pp. 171-179.

Bendon R, Siddigi J, de Courten-Myers G, Dignan P. (1987). *Recurrent developmental anomalies: 1. Syndrome with hidranencephaly with renal aplastic dysplasia, 2. Polyvalvular developmental heart defect*. Am J Genet Suppl, (January 1987), Vol. 3, pp. 357-365.

Bennet G, Bromley B, Banacerraf B. (1996). *Agenesis of the corpus callosum. Prenatal detection usually is not possible before 22 weeks gestation*. Radiology, (May 1996), Vol. 199, No. 2, pp. 447-450.

Bloom SL,SL, Bloom DD, Dellannebia C, Martin LB, Lucas MJ, Twickler DM. (1997). *The developmental outcome of the children with antenatal mild isolated ventriculomegaly: a retrospective analysis of 26 cases*. Obstet Gynecol, (July 1997), Vol. 90, No.1, pp. 93-97.

Bernard JP, Drummond CL, Zaarour P, Molho M, Ville Y. (2002). *A new clue to prenatal diagnosis of lobar holoprosencephaly: the abnormal pathway of the anterior cerebral artery crawling under the scul*. Ultrasound Obstet Gynecol, (June 2002), Vol. 19, No. 6, pp. 606-607.

Briellmann RS, Jackson GD, Torn-Broers Y, Berkovic SF. (1998). *Twins with different temporal lobe malformations: schizencephaly and arachnoid cyst*. Neuropediatrics, (December 1998), Vol. 29, No. 6, pp. 284-288.

Brunelle F. (1997). *Arteriovenous malformation of the vein of Galen in children*. Pediatr Radiol, (June 1997), Vol. 27, No. 6, pp. 501-513.

Byrd SE, Radkowski MA, Flannery A. (1990). *The clinical and radiological evaluation of absence of the corpus callosum* . Eur J Radiol, (January-February 1990), Vol. 10, No. 1, pp. 65-73.

Calabro F, Arcuri, T, Jinkins JR. (2000). *Blake's pouch cyst: an entity within Dandy-Walker continuum*. Neuroradiology, (April 2000), Vol.42, No. 4, pp. 290-295.

Carty H, Higham J & Crawford S, (Eds). (2001) *Pediatric ultrasound London*. Greenwich Medial Media Limited Publishers, ISBN 1900151170, London, UK.

Chapman S, Hockley AD. (1989). *Calcification of an aneurysm of the vein of Galen*. Pediatric Radiology, (September 1989), Vol.19, No. 8, pp. 541-542.

Chatzipapas IK, Whitlow BJ, Economides DL (1999). *The "Mickey Mouse" sign and the diagnosis of anencephaly in early pregnancy*. Ultrasound Obstet Gynecol, (March 1999), Vol. 13, No. 3, pp. 196-199.

Chavhan GB, Parra DA, Mann A, Navarro OM. (2008). *Normal Doppler spectral waveforms of major pediatric vessels: Specific patterns*. Radio Graphics, (May-June 2008), Vol. 28, No. 3, pp. 691-706.

Cheung YF, Lam PK, Yeung CY. (1994). *Early postnatal cerebral Doppler changes in relation to birth weight*. Early Hum Dev, (April 1994), Vol. 30, No. 1, pp. 57-66.

Cho FN, Kan YY, Chen SN, Lee teC, Hsu Tj, Hsu PH. (2005). *Prenatal diagnosis of cyclopia and proboscis in a fetus with normal chromosome at 13 WG by three-dimensional transabdominal sonography*. Prenat Diagn, (November 2005), Vol. 25, No. 11, pp. 1059-1060.

Couture AP. (2001). *Normal neonatal brain: colour Doppler and pulsed Doppler.* In: *Transfrontanellar Doppler imaging in neonates,* Couture A, Veyrac C, (Eds), 9-90, Springer Publishers, ISBN 3-5405-6463-6, Heidelberg , Germany.

D'Addario V, Pinto V, Del Bianco A, Di Naro E, Tartagni M, Miniello G, Serio G. (2001). *The clivus-supraoccipit angle: a useful measurement to evaluate the shape and size of the fetal posterior fossa and to diagnose Chiari II malformation.* Ultrasound Obstet Gynecol, (August 2001), Vol. 18, No. 2, pp. 146-149.

Davila-Gutierrez G. (2002). *Agenesis and dysgenesis of the corpus callosum.* Semin pediatr neurol, (December 2002), Vol. 9, No. 4, pp. 292-301.

Dean LM, Taylor GA. (1995). *The intracranial venous system in infants: normal and abnormal findings on duplex and color Doppler sonography.* Am J Roentgenol, (January 1995), Vol.164, No. 1, pp.151-156.

Deeg KH, Rupprecht T. (1989). *Pulsed Doppler sonographic measurement of normal values for the flow velocities in the intracranial arteries of healthy newborns.* Pediatr Radiol (April 1989), Vol. 19, No. 2, pp. 71–78.

Denis D, Chateil JF, Brun M, Brissaud O, Tontan D, Flurin V, Pedespan JM. (2000). *Schizencephaly: clinical and imaging features in 30 infantile cases.* Brain Development, (December 2000), Vol. 22, No. 8, pp. 475-483.

Dixon A. (1988), *Hidranencephaly.* Radiography, (January-February 1988), Vol. 54, No. 613, pp. 12-3.

Edison R, Muenke M. (2003). *The interplay of genetic and environmental factors in craniofacial morphogenesis: choloprosencephaly and the role of cholesterol.* Congenit Anom, (March 2003), Vol. 43, No. 1, pp.1-21.

Elbers SE, Furness ME. (1999). *Resolution of presumed arachnoid in utero.* Ultrasound Obstet Gynecol, (November 1999), Vol.14, No. 5, pp. 353-355.

Fong KW, Ghai S, Toi A, Blaser S, Winsor EJ, Chitayat D. (2004). *Prenatal ultrasound findings lissencephaly associated with Miller-Dieker syndrome and comparison with pre- and postnatal magnetic resonance imaging.* Ultrasound Obstet Gynecol, (December 2004), Vol. 24, No. 7, pp. 716-723.

Fransen E, Vits L, Van Camp G, Willems PJ. (1996). *The clinical spectrum of mutations in L1, a neuronal cell adhesion molecule.* Am J Med Genet, (July 1996), Vol. 64, No. 1, pp. 73-77.

Gaglioti P, Danelon D, Bontempo S, Mombro M, Cardaropoli S, Tordos T. (2005). *Fetal cerebral ventriculomegaly: outcome in 176 cases* (25) Ultrasound Obstet Gynecol, (April 2005), Vol. 25, No. 4, pp. 372-377.

Garel C, Chantrel E, Brisse H, Elmaleh M, Luton D, Oury J, Sebag G, Hassan M. (2001). *Fetal cerebral cortex: normal gestation landmarks identified using prenatal MR Imaging.* Am J Neuroradiol, (January 2001), Vol. 22, No. 1, pp. 184-189.

Goodwin L, Quisling RG. (1983). The neonatal cisterna magna: ultrasonic evaluation. Radiology, (December 1983), Vol. 149, No. 3, pp. 691-695.

Goodyear PW, Bannister CM, Russell S, Rimmer S. (2001). *Outcome in prenatally diagnosed fetal agenesis of corpus callosum.* Fetal Diagn Ther, (May-June 2001), Vol. 16, No. 3, pp. 139-145.

Graham E, Duhl A, Ural S, Allen M, Blakemore K, Witter F. (2001). The degree of antenatal ventriculomegaly is related to pediatric neurogical morbidity. J Matern Fetal Med, (August 2001), Vol.10, No. 4, pp. 258-263.

Granata T, Farina L, Faiella A, Cardini R, D'Incerti L, Boncinelli E, Battaglia G. (1997). *Familial schizencephaly associated with EMX2 mutation.* Neurology, (May 1997), Vol. 48, No. 5, pp. 1403-1406.

Griffiths P, Paley M & Whitby E, (Eds), (2006). *Imaging the central nervous system of the fetus and neonate*. Taylor and Francis Group Publishers, ISBN-13: 978-0-8247-2856-4, New York, USA.

Guerrini R, Carrozzo R. (2001). *Epilepsy and genetic malformations of the cerebral cortex*. Am J Med Genet, (Summer 2001), Vol. 106, No. 2, pp. 160-173.

Hanigan W, Aldrich W. (1998). *MRI and evoked potentials in a child with hidranencephaly*. Pediatric Neurol, (May-June 1988) Vol. 4, No. 3, pp. 185-187.

Hayashi N, Tsutsusumi Y, Barkovich AJ. (2002). Morphological features and associated anomalies of schizencephaly in the clinical population: detailed analysis of MR images. Neuroradiology, (May 2002), Vol. 44, No. 5, pp. 418-427.

Hetts SW, Sherr EH, Chao S, Gobuty S, Barkovich AJ. (2006). *Anomalies of the corpus callosum: An MR analysis of the phenotypic spectrum of associated malformations*. AJR, (November 2006), Vol.187, No. 5, pp. 1343-1348.

Hirohata M, Matsua H, Miyagi J, Kajihara K, Shigemori M, Kuramoto S. (1992). Interhemispheric arachnoid cyst; report of three cases. No Shinkei Geka, (June 1992), Vol. 20, No. 6, pp,701-705.

Iannetti P, Nigro G, Spalice A, Faiella A, Boncinelli E. (1998). *Cytomegalovirus infection and schizencephaly: case reports*. Ann Neurol, (January 1998), Vol. 43, No. 1, pp.123-127.

Kenwick S, Jouet M, Donnai D. (1996). *X-linked hydrocephalus and MASA syndrome*. Am J Med Genet, (January 1996), Vol. 33, No. 1, pp. 59-65.

Klein O, Pierre-Kahn A, Boddaert N, Parisot D, Brunelle F.(2003). Dandy-Walker malformation: prenatal diagnosis and prognosis. Childs Nerv Syst, (August 2003), Vol. 19, No. 7-8, pp. 484-489.

Lam YH, Tang MH. (2000). *Serial sonographic features of a fetus with hydranencephaly from 11 weeks to term*. Ultrasound Obste gynecol, (July 2000), Vol. 16, No. 1, pp. 77-79.

Levenet RJ. (2005). *Genotype-phenotype correlation in lissencephaly and subcortical band heterotopia: The key questions answered*, J Child Neurol, (April 2005), Vol. 20, No. 4, pp. 307-312.

Liang JS, Lee WT, Peng SS, Yu TW, Shen, YZ. (2002). *Schizencephaly: correlation between clinical and neuroimaging features*. Acta Paediatr Taiwan, (July-August 2002), Vol. 43, No. 4, pp. 208-213.

London DA, Caroll BA, Enzmann DR. (1980). *Sonography of ventricular size and germinal matrix haemorrhage in premature infants*. AJR, (September 1980), Vol. 135, No. 3, pp. 559-564.

Meizner I, Elchalal U. (1996). *Prenatal sonographic diagnose of anterior fossa porencephaly*. J Clin Ultrasound, (February 1996), Vol. 24, No. 2, pp. 96-99.

Mercier A, Eurin D, Mercier PY, Verspyck E, Marpeau L, Marret S. (2001). *Isolated mild fetal cerebral ventriculomegaly: a retrospective analysis of 26 cases*. Prenat Diagn, (July 2001), Vol. 21, No. 7, pp. 589-595.

Montenegro MA, Guareiro MM, Lopes-Cendes I, Guerreiro CA, Cendes F. (2002). *Interrelationship of genetics and prenatal injury in the genesis of malformations of cortical development*. Arch Neurol, (July 2002) Vol. 59, No. 7, pp. 1147-1153.

Muenke M, Beachey PA. (2000). *Genetics of ventral forebrain development and holoprosencephaly*. Curr Opin Genet Dev, (June 2000), Vol. 10, No. 3, pp. 262-269.

Nakamura Y, Mizukawa K, Yamamoto K, Nagashima T. (2001). *Endoscopic treatment for a huge neonatal prepontine-suprasellar arachnoid cyst: a case report*. Pediatr Neurosurg, (October 2001), Vol. 35, No. 4, pp. 220-224.

Nelson MD Jr, Maher K, Gilles FH. (2004). *A different approach to cysts on the posterior fossa.* Pediatr Radiol, (Septmber 2004), Vo. 34, No. 9, p. 720-732.

Nikas DC, Proctor MR, Scott RM. (1999). *Spontaneous thrombosis of vein of Galen aneurismal malformation.* Peditar Neurosurg, (July 1999), Vol. 31, No. 1, pp. 33-39.

Oh KY, Kennedy AM, Frias AE Jr, Byrne JLB. (2005). *Fetal schizencephaly: Pre- and Postnatal Imaging with a Review of the Clinical Manifestations.* RadioGraphic, (May-June 2005), Vol. 25, No. 3, pp. 647-657.

Preebles DM. (1998). *Holoprosencephaly.* Prenat Diagn, (May 1998), Vol.18, No. 5, pp. 477-480.

Penny SM. (2006). *Agenesis of the corpus callosum: neonatal sonographic detection.* Radiol Technol , (September-October 2006), Vol. 78, No. 1, pp. 14-18.

Pilu G, Falco P, Gabrielli S, Perolo A, Sandri R, Bovicelli L. (1999). *The clinical significance of fetal isolated cerebral borderline ventriculomegaly: report of 31 and review of the literature.* Ultrasound Obstet Gynecol, (November 1999), Vol. 14, No. 5, pp. 320–326.

Pilu G, Hobbins JC. (2002). *Sonography of fetal cerebrospinal anomalies.* Prenat Diagn, (April 2002), Vol. 22, No. 4, pp. 321-330.

Qusling RG, Reeder JD, Setzer ES, Kaude JV. (1983). *Temporal comparative analysis of computed tomography with ultrasound for intracranial haemorrhage in premature infants.* Neuroradiology, (February 1983), Vol. 24, No. 4, pp. 205-211.

Raybaud CA, Strother CM, Hald JK. (1989). *Aneurysms of the vein of Galen: embryonic considerations and anatomical features relating to the pathogenesis of the malformation.* Neuroradiology, (March 1989), Vol. 31, No. 2, pp. 109-128.

Renier D, Sainte-Rose C, Pierre-Kahn A, Firsch JF. (1988). *Prenatal hydrocephalus: outcome and prognosis.* Child Nerv Syst, (August 1988), Vol. 4, No.4, pp. 213-222.

Riccabona M, Nelson TR, Witzer C, Resch B, Pretorius DP. (2003). *Potential of three-dimensional ultrasound in neonatal and pediatric neurosonography.* Eur J Radiol, (September 2003), Vol. 13, No. 9, pp. 2082-2093

Robin ML, Filly RA, Goldstein RB. (1994). *The normal location of the fetal conus medullaris.* J Ultrasound Med, (July 1994), Vol 13, No. 7, pp. 541-546.

Roessler E, Muenke M. (1998). *Holoprosencephaly: a paradigm for the complex genetics of brain development.* J Inherit Metab Dis, (August 1998), Vol. 21, No. 5, pp. 481-497.

Romagnol C, Giannantonio C, Carolis MPD, Gallini F, Zecca E, Papacci P. (2006). *Neonatal color Doppler US study: Normal values of cerebral blood flow velocities in preterm infants in the first month of life.* Ultrasound in Med & Bio, (March 2006), Vol. 32, No. 3, pp. 321–331

Schell-Apacik CC, Wagner K, Bihler M, Ertl-Wagner B, Heinrich U, Klopocki E, Kalscheuer VM, Muenke M, von Voss H. (2008). *Agenesis and dysgenesis of the corpus callosum: clinical, genetics and neuroimaging findings in a series of 41 patients.* Am J Med Genet A, (October 2008), Vol. 146, No. 19, pp. 2501-2511.

Scher MS, Belfar H, Martin J, Painter MJ. (1991). *Destructive brain lesions of presumed fetal onset: antepartum causes of cerebral palsy.* Pediatrics, (November 1991), Vol. 88, No.5, pp. 898–906.

Schwanitz G, Schuler H, Gembruch U, Zerres K. (1993). *Chromosomal findings in fetuses with ultrasonographicly diagnosed ventriculomegaly.* Ann Genet, (January 1993), Vol. 36, No. 3, pp. 150-153.

Siegel MJ, Shackelford GD, Perlman JM, Fulling KH. (1984). *Hypoxic-ischemic encephalopathy in twin infants: Diagnosis and prognosis evaluated by ultrasound.* Radiol, (August 1984), Vol. 152, No.2, pp.395-399.

Signorelli M, Tiberti A, Valseriati D, Molin E, Cerri V, Groli C, Bianchi UA. (2004). *Width of the fetal lateral ventricular atrium between 10 and 12 mm: a simple variation of the norme.* Ultrasound Obstet Gynecol, (January 2004), Vol. 23, No. 1, pp 14–18.

Smith NC, Smith APM. (2006). *Detection of congenital fetal anomalies.* In; *Obstetric ultrasound made easy*, 2th, Smith NC, Smith APM, (Eds), 49-57, Churchill Livingstone, ISBN 044310055 1, Philadelphia, USA

Smith T, Tekes A, Boltshauser B, Huisman TAGM. (2008) *Comissural malformations: Beyond the corpus callosum.* J Neuroradiology, (December 2008), Vol. 35, No. 5, pp. 301-303.

Stevenson DA, Hart BL, Clericuzio CL. (2001). *Hydranencephaly in an infant vith vascular malformation.* Am J Med Genet, (December 2001), Vol. 15, No. 4, pp. 295-298.

Strand RD, Barnes PD, Young Pouissaint T, Estroff JA, Burrows PE. (1993). Cystic retrocerebellar malformation: unification of the Dandy-Walker complex and the Blake's pouch cyst. Pediatr Radiol, (July 1993), Vol. 23, No. 4, pp. 258-260.

Tang PH, Bartha AI, Norton ME, Barkovich AJ, Sherr EH, Glenn OA. (2009). *Agenesis of the corpus calosum: an MR imaging analysis of associated abnormalities in the fetus.* AJNR, (February 2009), Vol, 30, No. 2. Pp. 257-263.

Taylor M, David AS. (1998) *Agenesis of the corpus calosum: a United Kingdom series of 56 cases.* J Neurol Neurosurg Psychiatry, (January 1989), Vol. 64, No. 1, 131–134.

Toma P & Granata C. (2005). Brain sonography. In: Tortori-Donati P, Rossi A & Biancheri R, (Eds), *Pediatric neuroradiology brain*, 1115-1157, Springer, ISBN 3-540-41077-5, Berlin, Germany.

Trugg RD, Fletcher JC. (1989). *Anencephalic newborns: can organs be transplanted before brain death.* NEJM, (July 1989), Vol. 321, No. 2, pp. 88.

Vasiljevic B, Gojnic M, Maglajlic-Djukic S, Antonovic O. (2010). *Normal values of cerebral blood velocities in the neonates.* Srp Arh Celok Lek, (March-April 2010), Vol. 138, No. 3-4, pp. 186-91.

Vasiljevic B, Mglajlic-Djukic S, Stankovic S, Lutovac D, Gojnic M. (2011). Predictive value color Doppler ultrasonography for adverse neurodevelopment outcome in neonates with hypoxic ischemic encephalopathy. Vojnosanit Pregl, (October 2011), Vol. 68, No. 10, pp. 825-831.

Verloes A, Elmaleh M, Gonzales M, Laquerriere A, Gressens P. (2007). *Genetic and clinical aspects of lissencephaly.* Rev Neurol, Paris, (May 2007), Vol. 163, No. 5, pp. 533-547.

Vijayarghavan SB, Vijay S, Kala MR, Neha D. (2006). *Prenatal diagnosis of thrombosed aneurysm of vein of Galen.* Ultrasound Obstet Gynecol, (January 2006), Vol. 27, No. 1, pp. 81–83.

Volpe JJ. (2008) *Neural tube formation and prosencephalic development* In: *Neurology of newborn, 5th,* Volpe JJ, (Ed.), 3-43, *WB Sounders*, ISBN 978-1-4160-3995-2, Philadelphia, USA.

Volpe P, Campobasso G, De Robertis V, Rembouskos G. (2009). *Disorders in prosencephalic development.* Prenat Diagn, (April 2009), Vol. 29, No. 4, pp. 340-354.

Von Wezel-Meijler G, (Ed). (2007). *Neonatal cranial ultrasonography*, Springer, ISBN 978-3-540-69906-4, Berlin, Germany.

Wallis D, Muenke M. (2000). *Mutations in holoprosencephaly.* Hum Mutat, (Avgust 2000), Vol. 16, No. 2, pp. 99–108.

Whiteman VE, Reece EA. (1994). *Prenatal diagnosis of major congenital malformations.* Curr Opin Obst Gynae, (October 1994), Vol. 6, No. 5, pp. 459-467.

5

An Autopsy Case of Congenital Pulmonary Lymphangiectasis Masquerading as Pulmonary Interstitial Emphysema

Sohsuke Yamada and Yasuyuki Sasaguri
University of Occupational and Environmental Health
Kitakyushu

1. Introduction

Congenital pulmonary lymphangiectasis (CPL) is a rare and poorly documented disease of neonates, and is characterized by prominent and diffuse microcystic lymphatic dilation in the septal, subpleural and peribronchial tissue throughout both lungs. Although an accurate incidence of CPL is elusive, a previous autopsy study has suggested that approximately 1% of all infants stillborn or dead in the neonatal period have CPL (Laurence KM, 1955), and at least 30 and 130 cases of CPL have been reported in Japan and in the world, respectively. According to previous CPL reports, males are affected more than females, and there is no familial predisposition in most cases. However, a few cases have described an association with genetic disorders, such as Noonan, Down, Turner, and Fryns syndromes (Fryns JP & Moerman P, 1993; Jacquemont S et al., 2000). CPL is generally divided into two groups: primary (congenital) and secondary. In addition, Noonan classified CPL into three groups (Noonan JA et al., 1970): group 1 is characterized by generalized lymphangiectasis (lymphedema with intestinal lymphangiectasis) (Bellini C et al., 2001; Maclean JE et al, 2002); in group 2, CPL is caused by pulmonary venous hypertention or obstruction associated with surgery, radiation, infection, tumor, or cardiovascular anomalies including anomalous pulmonary venous drainage or cor triatriatum (Gilewski MK et al., 1996; Verlaat CWM et al., 1994); group 3 is due to a primary developmental defect of the pulmonary lymphatics (Huber A et al., 1991; Moerman P et al., 1993). Therefore, groups 1 and 3 of CPL are primary (congenital), and group 2 is secondary. In particular, group 3 CPL is characterized by severely disturbed pulmonary gas exchange and a poor prognosis (Hoehn T et al., 2006), and some reports have shown that neonates with group 3 CPL have lymphatic dilation in the lungs and multiple other organs, and pursue an adverse clinical course (Frank J et al., 1955; Hirano H et al., 2004; Mckendry JBJ et al., 1957). Because of the clinicopathological similarities between group 3 CPL and pulmonary interstitial emphysema (PIE), CPL tends to be misdiagnosed as PIE (Finder J & Steinfeld J, 2004; Xiao ZY et al., 2009). Although a conclusive diagnosis of CPL can only be made pathologically or by autopsy, CPL should be distinguished from PIE because of their distinct treatments and prognoses (Laurence KM, 1955; Finder J & Steinfeld J, 2004; Xiao ZY et al., 2009).

2. Case report

An autopsy case of CPL group 3 is described with a special reference to distinction from PIE.

2.1 Clinical summary

A male Japanese neonate was born at 34 weeks of gestation after the pregestational treatment for infertility and medication for mild amniorrhexis, and was the second child born to non-consanguineous parents. The parents' first baby weighed 3,276 g and was born at 40 weeks of spontaneous gestation 5 years before this case. The patient weighed about 2,300 g at birth, and his Apgar scores were 7 and 8 at 1 and 5 minutes, respectively. The amniotic fluid was clear, and the amount was approximately 400 mL. The placenta, weighing 460 g, had no remarkable features. However, he developed a severe moaning sound and dyspnea about 10 minutes after birth, in spite of artificial oxygenation. A chest X-ray film showed bilateral frosted glass-like infiltrates with an air bronchogram and an air leak (arrows) around the cardiac shadow, suggesting pneumomediastinum (Fig. 1).

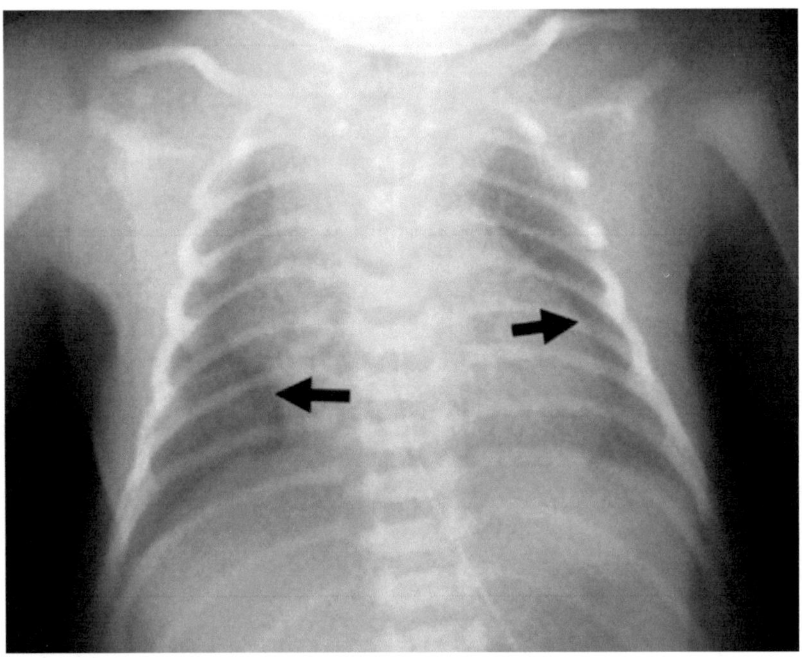

Fig. 1. Plain chest X-ray.

Despite artificial ventilation after intubation and surfactant substitution therapy, he died of hypoxemic respiratory failure 13 hours after birth due to persistent pneumomediastinum and bilateral pneumothorax, which were resistant to the puncture by thoracostomy tubes and the intravenous administration of dopamine and bicarbonate. The blood cell counts and values of blood biochemistry were within normal limits, except for a venous blood sample when breathing at 30% oxygen concentration in the incubator showing elevated partial pressure of carbon dioxide ($PaCO_2$) (70.7 mmHg), and decreased base excess (-7.4 mEq/L) and pH (7.145), indicating marked respiratory acidosis. An autopsy was performed approximately 3 hours after death.

2.2 Gross findings

At autopsy, the baby measured 45cm in height and weighed 2,328 g. An external examination showed no detectable anomalies or abnormalities except for several needle marks on the chest wall and the extremities. In an internal examination of the thoracic cavity (Fig. 2) there was a bilateral clear yellow pleural fluid (20 mL; 20 mL) without hemorrhage or chylothorax, and one cystic lesion was noted in the anterior mediastinum.

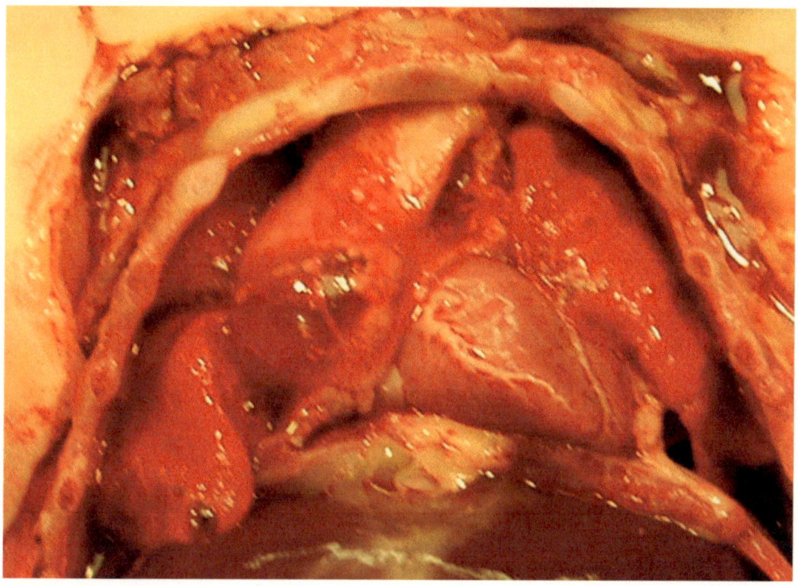

Fig. 2. An internal examination of the thoracic cavity.

In addition to the visceral pleura, both lungs demonstrated a network of dilated cystic spaces. The left and right lungs weighed 21 g and 23 g, respectively, and were firm in consistency. The cut surfaces of the congestive lungs also showed numerous cystic spaces ranging from about 1 to 2 mm in size in the surface visceral pleura as well as in the thickened interlobular septum and hilum, although the cystic changes were inconspicuous after formalin fixation. These findings were well recognized in a hematoxylin-eosin-stained scanning magnification of the lungs (Fig. 3).

The heart, weighing 18 g, showed no gross abnormalities. No specific findings were identified in the other internal organs or the brain, except for a clear yellow peritoneal fluid (150 mL).

2.3 Pathological findings

A histological examination of the lungs showed diffuse and marked lymphatic dilation in the peribronchial (Fig. 4A), subpleural, interlobular (Fig. 4B) and hilar areas.

The dilated lymphatic channels were invariably lined with flattened endothelium, which was immunohistochemically positive for D2-40 (Nichirei Bioscience Co., Tokyo, Japan, 1:1) (Fig. 5), CD31 (Dako Cytomation Co., Kyoto, Japan, 1:20) and CD34 (IMMUNOTECH, Marseille, France, 1:50).

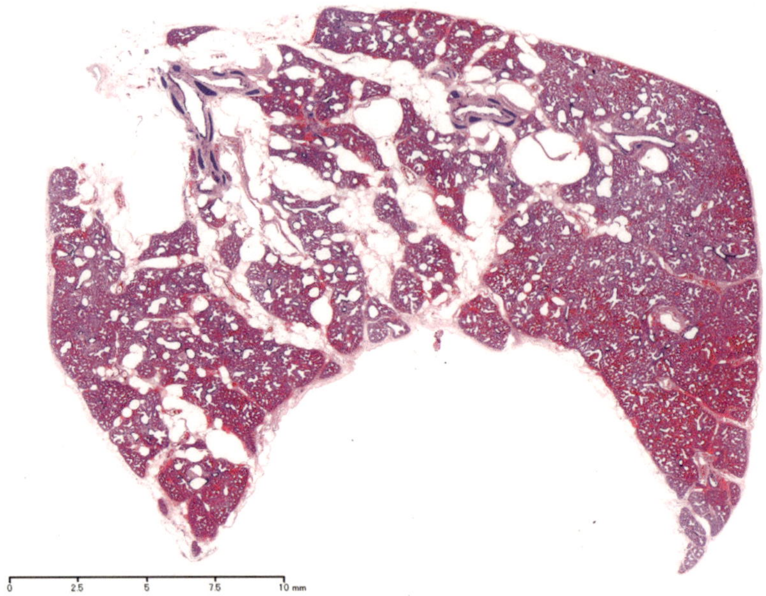

Fig. 3. Scanning magnification of the lung, right lower lobe.

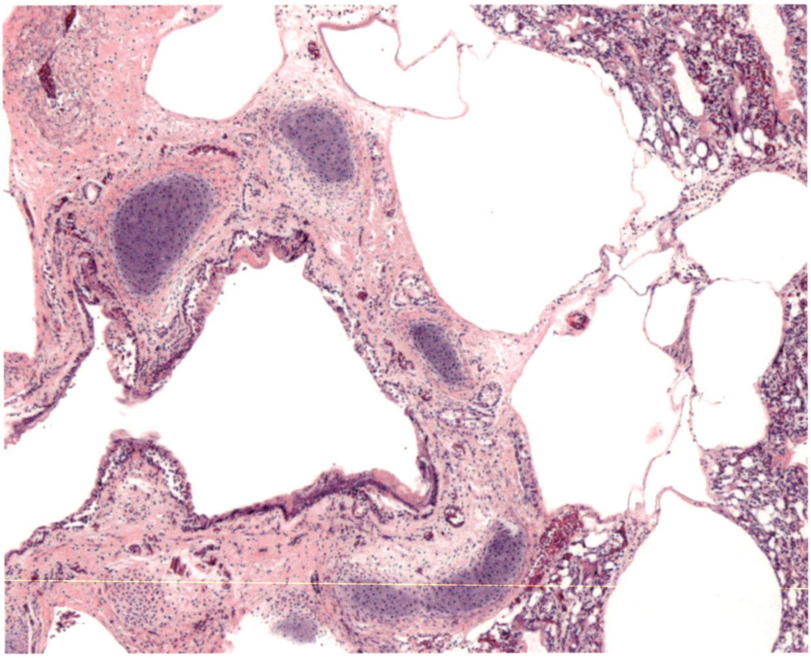

Fig. 4A. Histological finding of CPL (peribronchial).

No CD68-positive (Dako, 1:100) foreign-body type histiocytes were seen in these cystically-dilated lesions. Most of the mature-looking alveolar spaces were collapsed, and the alveolar walls were close to each other with frequent deposits of hyaline membrane along the bronchioli or alveolar ducts, accompanied by accumulated basophilic amorphous materials

(Fig. 6), which were negative for Kossa staining and probably derived from the necrotic bronchioloalveolar epithelium (Wigglesworth JS, eds., 1984).

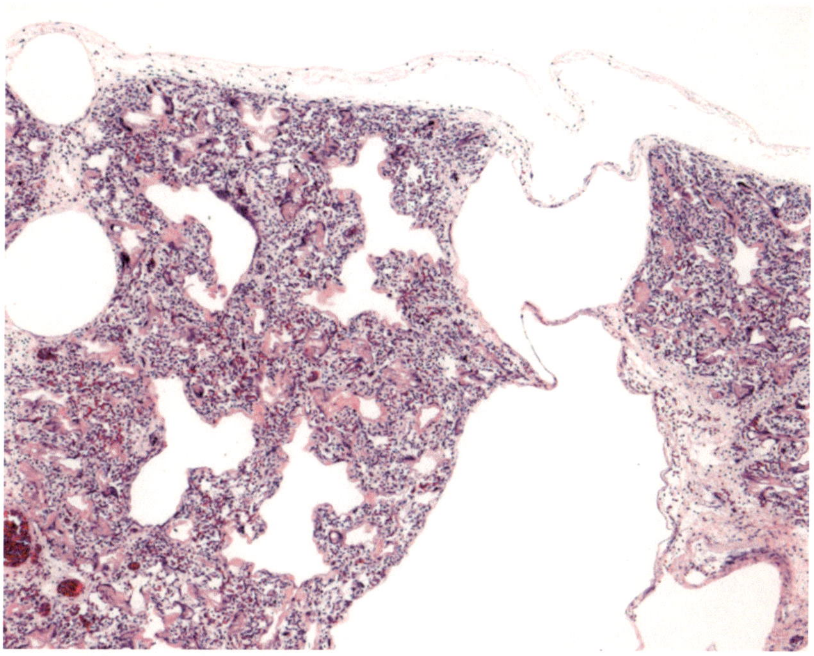

Fig. 4B. Histological finding of CPL (subpleural and interlobular).

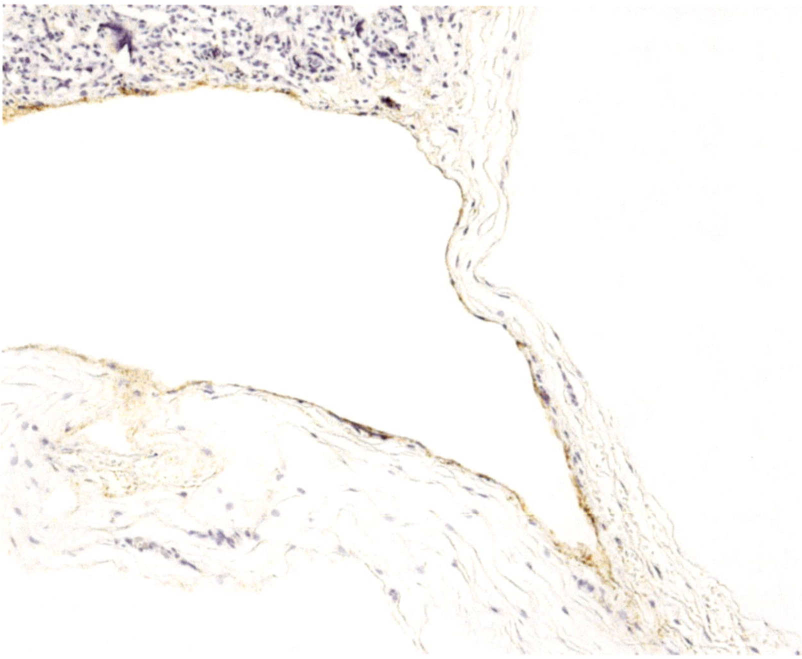

Fig. 5. Immunohistochemical finding of the dilated lymphatic channels.

Additionally, mild lymphangiectasis was found around the mediastinum including the thymus and the intra-abdominal organs such as the adrenal gland, kidney, pancreas, spleen, sigmoid colon, and abdominal aorta, all of which also lacked any foreign-body reaction. Pseudofollicular cysts were present in the definitive adrenal cortex (Fig. 7).

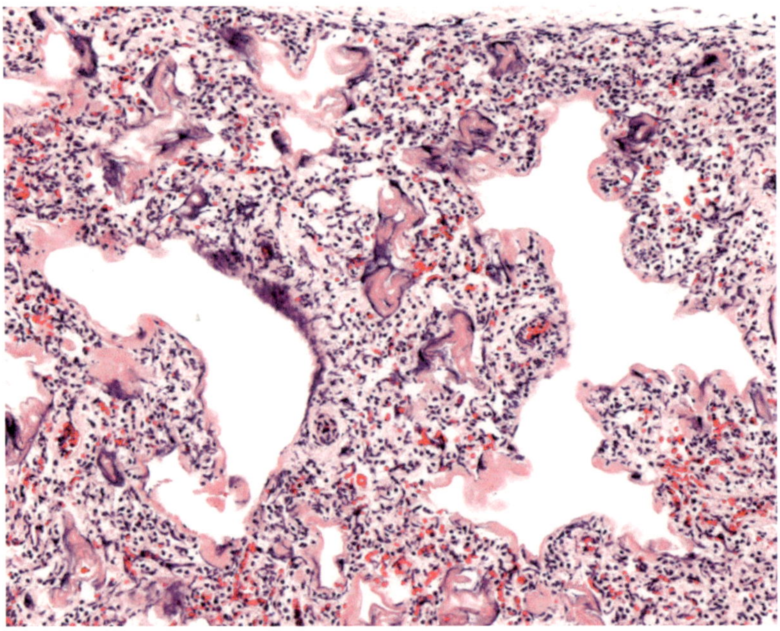

Fig. 6. Histological finding of the bronchioli to alveolar spaces.

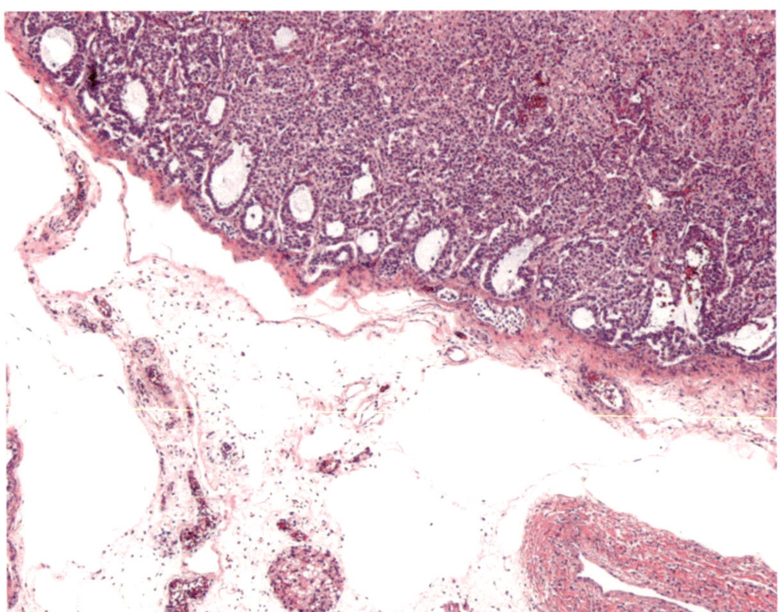

Fig. 7. Histological finding of the adrenal gland.

The diagnosis of CPL, a primary form, Noonan Group 3, was established based on these features.

2.4 Discussion

Congenital pulmonary lymphangiectasis (CPL) was first described by Virchow (Virchow R, 1856), demonstrating clinical manifestations of aggressive dyspnea after birth, cyanosis and death. The lungs of CPL show grossly dilated lymph channels beneath the pleura and in the variably thickened interlobular septa, and these dilated lymph vessels are also recognized in the subpleura, interlobular septa, and peribronchial tissue throughout both lungs microscopically. The mortality rate of neonatal CPL was considered to be nearly 100% more than 30 years ago. However, because neonatal care has advanced significantly since then, the outcome of the patients has improved, especially for those who present the symptoms after the neonatal period or for those belonging to Noonan classification group 1 or 2 (Hirano H et al., 2004; Moerman P et al., 1993). Nevertheless, Noonan group 3 CPL is usually associated with an adverse clinical course and high mortality. It is well known that group 3 CPL is due to a developmental error, probably resulting from a failure of pulmonary interstitial connective tissue to regress and leading to the dilation of pulmonary lymphatic vessels (Xiao ZY et al., 2009). This usually occurs after the 16th week of fetal life (Faul JL et al., 2000; Laurence KM, 1995), followed by insufficient dilatation of alveolar structures. These pathological changes might result in severe pulmonary symptoms (Janett SN et al., 1963), probably including those due to respiratory distress syndrome (RDS).

CPL is often difficult to differentiate from pulmonary interstitial emphysema (PIE) because of the clinicopathological similarities between these two diseases (Laurence KM, 1955; Finder J & Steinfeld J, 2004; Xiao ZY et al., 2009). PIE in the newborn is a frequent complication of RDS or hyaline membrane disease. The typical chest X-ray findings of PIE include multiple large cysts (0.8-3.0 cm) in a background of smaller cysts (0.2-0.4 cm) with uniform minute reticulogranular densities and abnormal airbronchograms caused by RDS (Stocker JT & Madewell JE, 1977). The X-ray in the current case showed bilateral frosted glass-like or cotton-like infiltrates with an air bronchogram and an air leak around the cardiac shadow due to RDS and pneumomediastinum, partly resembling the findings of PIE complicated by pneumomediastinum. Moreover, the patient suffered an uncontrollable bilateral pneumothorax after artificial ventilation was started. Therefore, a clinical distinction between these entities is not straightforward, and a definitive diagnosis of CPL can be made only by pathological examinations (Laurence KM, 1955; Finder J & Steinfeld J, 2004; Xiao ZY et al., 2009). The small cysts of PIE are invariably lined by mono- and multinucleated giant histiocytes displaying a foreign-body type reaction (Keeling JW, eds., 1993). In contrast, cysts in CPL are lined with flattened endothelium without evidence of aggregated histiocytes. Although this case demonstrated pneumothorax and pneumomediastinum, their etiological mechanisms are not easy to explain. However, the bilateral pneumothorax might have been caused by the artificial ventilation, which often results in air leak to the extra-airspaces, rather than by RDS itself. As to the pneumomediastinum prior to the ventilation and pneumothorax, a dilated lymphatic vessel might have been misunderstood as air leakage forming the persistent cystic lesion in the anterior mediastinum, in which, not only the immunohistochemical result of D2-40 showed positive-stainings, but also no giant cell reaction was identified. Furthermore, it is certain that RDS is sometimes accompanied by pulmonary lymphangiectasis, which might or might not lead to mediastinal lymphangiectasis, to a degree that renders its distinction from CPL difficult (Keeling JW, eds., 1993). However, in RDS, distended lymphatics are primarily interlobular in location, while in CPL they are also found in the subpleural and peribronchial areas and are wider in size, as in the present case. From these viewpoints, it is suggested that this pulmonary to mediastinal lymphangiectasis is caused by not only CPL, but also by RDS, although to a lesser degree.

Besides PIE, CPL should be distinguished from diffuse pulmonary lymphangiomatosis (DPL) (Hirano H et al., 2004; Bush JK et al., 1969; Brown M et al., 1999), because of their similar clinical manifestations and histological features. In addition, an immunohistochemical approach cannot differentiate between CPL and DPL, both of which share positive stainings for vimentin, CD31, CD34, factor VIII-related antigen, and D2-40. Histologically, DPL is characterized by an increased number of complex anastomosing lymphatic channels, in which variable dilation or expansion is a secondary phenomenon within the lungs and mediastinum, whereas in CPL the lymphatics are not increased in number and are relatively more regular in size and shape (Bush JK et al., 1969; Brown M et al., 1999; Hirano H et al., 2004; Moerman P et al., 1993). Based on these features, DPL could also be excluded in our case.

3. Conclusion

Herein was reported a neonate case of group 3 CPL with pathological findings of lymphangiectasis in or around multiple organs, including both lungs, the mediastinum, and those in the intra-abdominal cavity. Although PIE was considered an important differential diagnosis because of the overlapping clinicopathological features, a giant cell reaction surrounding the interstitial cystic lesions, a histological hallmark of PIE, was absent in the present case.

4. References

Bellini, C.; Bonioli, E., Josso, N., Belville, C., Mazzella, M., Costabel, S., Sementa, AR., Marino, CE., Tomà, P., Hennekam, RC. & Serra, G. (2001). Persistence of Mullerian derivatives and intestinal lymphangiectasis in two newborn brothers: confirmation of the urioste syndrome, *Am J Med Genet*, Vol.104, No.1, pp. 69-74.

Brown, M.; Pysher, T. & Coffin, CM. Lymphangioma and congenital pulmonary lymphangiectasis: a histologic, immunohistochemical, and clinicopathologic comparison. (1999). *Mod Pathol*, Vol.12, No.6, pp. 569-575.

Bush, JK.; McLean, RL. & Sieker, HO. Diffuse lung disease due to lymphangiomyoma. (1969). *Am J Med*, Vol.46, No.4, pp. 645-654.

Faul, JL.; Berry, GJ., Colby, TV., Ruoss, SJ., Walter, MB., Rosen, GD. & Raffin, TA. (2000). Thoracic lymphangiomas, lymphangiectasis, lymphangiomatosis, and lymphatic dysplasia syndrome. *Am J Respir Crit Care Med*, Vol.161, No.3, pp. 1037-1046.

Finder, J. & Steinfeld, J. Congenital pulmonary lymphangiectasia. *N Engl J Med*, 2004; Vol.350, No.9, pp. 948.

Frank, J.; Piper, PG. & Wis, M. Congenital pulmonary cystic lymphangiectasis. (1959). *J Am Med Assoc*, Vol.171, pp. 1094-1098.

Fryns, JP. & Moerman, P. 46,XY/46,XX mosaicism and congenital pulmonary lymphangiectasis with chylothorax. (1993). *Am J Medical Genet*, Vol.47, No.6, pp. 934-935.

Gilewski, MK.;, Statler, CC., Kohut, G. & Toriello, HV,. Congenital pulmonary lymphangiectasia, and other anomalies in a child: provisionally unique syndrome? (1996). *Am J Med Genet*, Vol.66, No.4, pp. 438-440.

Hirano, H.; Nishigami, T., Okimura, A., Nakasho, K. & Uematsu, K. Autopsy case of congenital pulmonary lymphangiectasis. (2004). *Pathol Int*, Vol.54, Vol.7, pp. 532-536.

Hoehn, T.; William, M., McPhaden, AR., Stannigel, H., Mayatepek, E. & Wadsworth, RM. Endothelial, inducible and neuronal nitric oxide synthase in congenital pulmonary lymphangiectasia. (2006). *Eur Respir J*, Vol.27, No.6, pp. 1311-1315.

Huber, A.; Schranz, D., Blaha, I., Schmitt-Mechelke, T. & Schumacher, R. Congenital pulmonary lymphangiectasia. (1991). *Pediatr Pulmonol*, Vol.10, No.4, pp. 310-313.

Jacquemont, S.; Barbarot, S., Boceno, M., Stalder, JF. & David, A. (2000). Familial congenital pulmonary lymphangiectasia, non-immune hydrops fetalis, facial and lower limb lymphedema: confirmation of Njolstad's report. *Am J Med Genet*, Vol.93, No.4, pp. 264-268.

Janett, SN.; Webster, I. & Braudo, JL. Congenital dilatation of the pulmonary lymphatics. (1963). *Pediatrics*, Vol.31: 416-425.

Keeling, JW., eds. (1993) *Fetal and Neonatal Pathology. 2nd ed.* London: Springer-Verlag.

Laurence KM. Congenital pulmonary cystic lymphangiectasis (1955). *J Pathol Bacteriol*, 1955; Vol.70, No.2, pp. 325-333.

Maclean, JE.; Cohen, E. & Weinstein, M. Primary intestinal and thoracic lymphangiectasia: a response to antiplasmin therapy. (2002). *Pediatrics*, Vol.109, No.6, pp. 1117-1180.

Mckendry, JBJ.; Lindsay, WK. & Gerstein, MC. Congenital defect of lymphatics in infancy. (1957). *Pediatrics*, Vol.19, No.1, pp. 21-35.

Moerman, P.; Vandenberghe, K., Devlieger, H., Van Hole, C., Fryns, JP. & Lauweryns, JM. Congenital pulmonary lymphangiectasis with chylothorax: a heterogeneous lymphatic vessel abnormality. (1993). *Am J Med Genet*, Vol.47, No.1, pp. 54-58.

Noonan, JA.; Walters, LR. & Reeves, JT. Congenital pulmonary lymphangiectasis. (1970). *Am J Dis Child*, Vol.120, No.4, pp. 314-319.

Stocker, JT. & Madewell, JE. Persistent interstitial pulmonary emphysema: another complication of the respiratory distress syndrome. (1977). *Pediatrics*, Vol.59, No.6, pp. 847-857.

Verlaat, CWM.; Peters, HM., Semmekrot, BA. & Wiersma-van Tilburg JM. Congenital pulmonary lymphangiectasia, presenting as a unilateral hyperlucent lung. (1994). *Eur J Pediatr*, Vol.153, No.3, pp. 202-205.

Virchow, R. (1856). *Gesammelte Abhandlungen zur wissenschaftlichen Medicin.* Frankfort: Meidinger, pp. 982.

Wigglesworth, JS., eds. (1984). *Perinatal Pathology. 1st ed.* Philadelphia: W.B. Saunders Company.

Xiao, ZY; Tao, Y., Tang, XY., Chen, GJ. & Guo, L. Congenital pulmonary lymphangiectasis. (2009). *World J Pediatr*, Vol.5, No.1, pp. 68-70.

6

Assisted Reproductive Technology and Congenital Malformations

Johanna A. Reed and Alastair G. Sutcliffe
University College London
United Kingdom

1. Introduction

Assisted reproductive technology (ART) encompasses all medical intervention used to assist people becoming parents, mainly but not solely as a result of infertility. In vitro fertilisation (IVF) is the cornerstone of ART. It involves stimulating the ovaries, retrieving and culturing oocytes which are then inseminated with capacitated spermatozoa. The embryo is cultured and transferred into the uterus. The first successful IVF pregnancy came to term in 1978. Since then numbers have rapidly increased and it now accounts for nearly 2% of births in the UK and more than 4 million worldwide (Human Fertilisation and Embryology Authority, 2011; ICMART, 2008).

There has always been concern about the possibility of an increased rate of congenital malformations in children conceived using ART. Analysis of early longitudinal data from Australia showed a higher rate of transposition of the great arteries and spina bifida in individuals conceived by IVF than expected (Lancaster, 1987). In IVF, sperm and eggs are removed from their normal environment and subject to altered hormones, handling and culture media. Newer techniques such as Intracytoplasmic sperm injection (ICSI) and preimplantation genetic diagnosis (PGD) are even more invasive, potentially leaving the developing embryo at greater risk of malformation. Major malformations are usually defined as those which generally cause functional impairment, other conditions are considered to be minor anomalies (Holmes, 1976).

Studying ART outcomes has proved difficult. Initial studies were small and there was a confounding high incidence of multiple births. Methodological pitfalls included difficulty finding adequate control groups as the ART population differs from the general population. The underlying cause of infertility might itself lead to pregnancy loss and congenital malformation and surveillance is often more rigorous following ART pregnancies (Simpson, 1996).

As more babies are born as a result of these techniques, there is more data available regarding the outcomes, and increasing evidence that there is a slightly higher risk of congenital malformations than following spontaneous conception. This chapter begins with an overview of ART and then moves on to discuss associated malformations and potential mechanisms. It was produced following a Medline search using the MeSH terms 'fertilisation in vitro' AND 'congenital malformation'. References from articles selected were reviewed to find additional articles.

2. Assisted reproductive technology

The term assisted reproductive technology (ART) covers a range of techniques to enable people to have children who wouldn't otherwise be able to. It can be used to assist fertilisation in vivo with ovulation induction, intra uterine insemination and gamete intrafallopian transfer (GIFT). When in vivo fertilisation is not possible in-vitro fertilisation (IVF) is described above.

Intracytoplasmic sperm injection (ICSI) was initially used where sperm are unable to fertilise the egg. A single sperm is selected based on morphological characteristics and injected into the oocyte cytoplasm. It was first used in 1992 (Palermo et al., 1992) and its high success rate has led it to be used in many centres for all cause infertility. If sperm can not be produced without medical intervention it can be collected directly from the epididymis by percutaneous epididymal sperm aspiration (PESA) or from the testicles, by testicular sperm aspiration (TESA). It is also possible to remove tiny quantities of testicular tissue from which sperm can be extracted using testicular sperm extraction (TESE). As only small numbers of sperm are produced by these methods, ICSI is then used to achieve fertilisation.Âă

Preimplantation genetic screening or diagnosis (PGS/PGD) is used in families known to have a genetic disease or with previous recurrent miscarriages. It is used to select either embryos without disease or âĂŸsaviour siblingsâĂŹ where HLA matched cells could be used as treatment for an already affected individual (Rubio, 2010). Embryos are produced by IVF or ICSI and then one or two cells are taken from the embryo by a trained embryologist at day two or three and tested for the features required. Acceptable embryos are transferred to the uterus to allow them to develop and suitable remaining unaffected embryos can be cryopreserved for later use. Embryos which are affected by the condition are allowed to perish.

Eggs, ovarian tissue, sperm and embryos can be cryopreserved for use in the future. Embryos are usually from IVF cycles, gametes are stored to preserve fertility for example while undergoing treatment for cancer. With an increase in single embryo transfer, more embryos are being frozen and this can be done at several stages with potential for differing outcomes. Egg cryopreservation is the most recent possibility as it has been difficult to develop techniques to prevent eggs bursting.

3. Adverse perinatal outcomes

Initial longitudinal studies of IVF in England (MRC Working Party on Children Conceived by In Vitro Fertilisation, 1990) and Australia (Australian in vitro fertilisation collaborative group, 1985) showed poor outcomes for IVF infants with significant low birth weight and prematurity. These risks have subsequently been confirmed by multiple studies and systematic reviews (Hansen et al., 2005; 2002; Helmerhorst et al., 2004; Jackson et al., 2004; Schieve et al., 2007; 2002).

The most well documented risk of ART is multiple births. Assisted conception accounts for 1.7% of all births but 21% of multiple births in the UK (Human Fertilisation and Embryology Authority, 2011). Higher order births are more likely to be born preterm, have a lower birth weight and have congenital malformations. Single embryo transfer is now promoted which has reduced these complications. Despite this ART children still have a higher perinatal morbidity and mortality than matched controls (Al-Fifi et al., 2009; Helmerhorst et al., 2004). A systematic review found that for singletons the relative risk of a very preterm birth (<32 weeks) was 3.27 (95% CI 2.03 -5.28) after assisted conception (Helmerhorst et al., 2004).

4. Congenital malformations

A large number of studies have been conducted looking at malformations in ART conceived children. Couples using ART differ from the general population in several ways and results have been particularly complicated by difficulty finding adequate control groups. Typically they are older, have a higher socioeconomic status and are infertile. The underlying cause of infertility might itself lead to malformation and it is difficult to find appropriate infertile controls who have spontaneously conceived. It may be that couples are less likely to terminate pregnancies conceived by IVF thus increasing the rate of children born with congenital malformations. In early studies ART offspring were rigorously examined and malformation rates then compared to the general population who may have only undergone superficial examination and malformations may not have been recorded appropriately. Many studies only examined children for abnormalities at birth when fewer congenital anomalies can be identified compared to at 6 months of age. Birth defects should be assessed without knowledge of conception status but it has been shown that paediatricians are relatively good at determining this from other cues (Ludwig, Katalinic, Entenmann, Thyen, Sutcliffe, Diedrich & Ludwig, 2009). There are few studies looking at ART outcomes in people using the techniques for reasons other than infertility.

It is possible that ART may predispose to only certain types of malformations. The initial Australian study suggested a link with cardiac and neural tube defects (Lancaster, 1987). An early study of all infants born in Sweden after IVF, 1982âĂŞ1997 (n = 9111) found a 3-fold excess risk of neural tube defects, alimentary atresia and omphalocele (Ericson & Källén, 2001). It found an increased risk for hypospadias after ICSI but not after standard IVF. In a follow up study this group continued to find an increased risk of neural tube defects, choanal atresia and alimentary tract atresia in this population (**?**). Further work in Australia found a specific association between ART and 'blastogenesis birth defects' arising in the first 4 weeks of pregnancy such as abdominal wall defects, vertebral segmentation defects, tracheoesophageal fistula, diaphragmatic defects, neural tube defects, anal atresia and renal agenesis. They were present in 1 in 160 ART pregnancies compared with 1 in 400 controls (Halliday et al., 2010).

A recent study from Paris found cases of congenital heart disease were more likely to have been conceived using ART (Tararbit et al., 2011). ART was specifically associated with significant increases in the odds of malformations of the outflow tracts and ventriculoarterial connections (adjusted OR 1.7, 95% CI 1.2âĂŞ2.4) and of cardiac neural crest defects and double outlet right ventricle (adjusted OR 1.7, 95% CI 1.1âĂŞ2.7) (Tararbit et al., 2011). A retrospective cohort study again found a higher rate of cardiovascular malformations in infants conceived by ART than controls (Wen et al., 2010). An American study of infants with birth defects found more infants had been conceived by ART and a specific association with septal heart defects (Reefhuis et al., 2009). Fetal echocardiography did not find an increase of congenital heart defects above the general population but it did find higher rates in twin pregnancies compared to singletons which may contribute to earlier findings (Bahtiyar et al., 2010).

Several studies have found an increased rate of cerebral palsy in children born following IVF (Hvidtjørn et al., 2010; 2006; Lidegaard et al., 2005; Zhu et al., 2010). In some cases this has been accounted for by the high rate of multiple births and preterm delivery (Hvidtjørn et al., 2010; 2006). Some have found the risk remains increased when accounting for these confounders (Lidegaard et al., 2005; Zhu et al., 2010; **?**).

Looking at malformations overall Rimm et al. performed a meta-analysis of 19 controlled studies comparing major malformation rates in IVF and ICSI children with spontaneously conceived children (Rimm et al., 2004). They found an odds ratio for major malformations of 1.29 (95%CI 1.01-1.67) in children conceived by IVF/ICSI. There was no significant difference in malformation rates in individuals conceived by IVF compared to ICSI. There was a lot of variation in major malformation rates between studies. The odds ratio for malformations was higher in singletons compared to multiple births, probably because of the increase in monozygotic twins with a higher rate of malformations after spontaneous conception. There were many problems identified with the studies used in this meta- analysis. Most used inappropriate groups of healthy controls which often did not control for the older age and fertility problems of parents using ART. There was no distinguishing if cryopreservation had been used.

Overall, meta-analysis has shown a 40-50% increased rate of major malformations following ART (Hansen et al., 2005; Lie et al., 2005; Rimm et al., 2004). A recent update (Rimm et al., 2011) included an augmented calculation of the contribution of infertility (Zhu et al., 2006). This found ART does not increase the risk of major malformations as much as previously reported when subfertile couples are used as controls suggesting a proportion of the increased risk of congenital malformations following IVF is due to the underlying subfertility rather than ART per se.

5. Mechanisms leading to congenital malformations in ART children

5.1 Point mutations

In very rare cases a mutation can be found which has shown variable expression, causing infertility in the parent and a more apparent congenital malformation in the offspring.

5.1.1 IHH and SOX2 mutations

A mother with idiopathic hypogonadotrophic hypogonadism had given birth to two children following ovulation induction. One had anopthalmia and one had unilateral micropthalmia (Stark et al., 2011). All three were subsequently found to be carriers of a SOX2 mutation. Studies appeared to show the mother carried a lower level of DNA with this mutation but they were unable to determine if she was a mosaic.

5.1.2 Cystic fibrosis

Previous studies have shown CFTR mutations in a significant proportions in azoospermic (31%) and oligospermic (22%) men (Gallati et al., 2009). If the mother is also heterozygous for a CFTR mutation the offspring may have more manifestations of cystic fibrosis.

5.2 Chromosomal abnormalities

Chromosomal abnormalities are an uncommon cause of malformations following ART. About 4.6% of infertile men with with oligospermia and 13.7% with aspermia and have a coexistent chromosome abnormality which is most frequently a deletion in the long arm of the Y chromosome (Foresta & Ferlin, 2001; Vicdan et al., 2004). A recent study found 4.3% (5/115) azoospermic men had a karyotype abnormality, 80% of these were Kleinfelters syndrome (Koşar et al., 2010). Most centres now perform a karyotype as part of a basic infertility screen.

5.2.1 Ring Y

A case has been reported of an infant conceived by ICSI with ambiguous genitalia (Spinner et al., 2008). The father had presented with infertility and oligospermia. The child's karyotype was 47,XXr(Y)[10]/46,XX[40]. The ring Y chromosome was inherited from the father. A simillar case from an oligospermic father following ICSI has been reported previously, in a child with a 45,X/46,Xr(Y) mosaicism (Bofinger et al., 1999).

5.2.2 Aneuploidy

Cases have been reported of an unusual karyotype in association with trisomy 21 in individuals conceived by IVF with embryo cryopreservation. One report described a mosaic where one cell line contained an additional copy of chromosome 21 as part of a Robertsonian translocation and the other cell line contained a ring chromosome 21 (Guran et al., 2010).

An evaluation of products of conception following miscarriage in ART pregnancies or spontaneous conception in subfertile couples showed an abnormal karyotype in 63.2% cases after ART and in 71.5% after natural conception in subfertile couples.41 Overall 60% of such abortuses would be expected to have an abnormal karyotype. Only 10 ICSI-TESE cases were analysed, and there was a discrepancy between chromosome abnormalities detected in this group (80%) compared to ICSI (61.5%). 50% showed triploid/tetraploid karyotypes, when in the other groups polyploidy did not exceed 17.5%. Although numbers are very small authors hypothesize that the use of immature testicular spermatozoa confers a higher risk of cytogenetically abnormal conceptions (Bettio et al., 2008).

5.3 Epigenetic abnormalities

Imprinted genes are those where only one allele is normally expressed, according to the parent of origin (Amor & Halliday, 2008). About 1% of human genes are thought to be imprinted, typically paternally expressed genes promote growth whereas maternally expressed genes suppress growth. The signal for this origin specific expression is an epigenetic change in the form of methylation and histone modification, changing the structure of the DNA rather than the sequence. With each generation the imprinted signal is erased and re-establised during gametogenesis.

Several mechanisms can lead to errors of imprinting, some of which cause recognised syndromes. There may be a mutation in one allele of an imprinted gene which prevents its expression or a larger deletion encompasing a whole gene or its imprinting control centre. A child can inherit two copies of a chromosome from one parent, uniparental disomy. An alternative mechanism is an epigenetic abnormality, for example affecting methylation. For each of the recognised imprinting syndromes the rates with which each mechanism accounts for cases differs.

There have been reports of unexpectedly raised rates of imprinting disorders in children born after assisted conception. Analysis indicates that imprinting defects in these individuals are largely due to epigenetic defects, specifically aberrant DNA methylation (Bahtiyar et al., 2010; Odom & Segars, 2010). It is hypothesised that the erasure and reestablishment of the imprinting signal may be disrupted by some forms of ART. The demands placed on the embryo by ART may induce adaptations in foetal epigenetic patterns eventually leading to such imprinting disorders. Indeed, altered epigenetic patterns have been found in assisted conception embryos, cord blood and placenta (Turan et al., 2010).

Loss or gain of the epigenetic signal can occur on either the maternal or paternal allele but in most reported cases affecting ART children the problem is hypomethylation on the maternal allele (Amor & Halliday, 2008). There is no evidence other mechanisms such as large deletions or duplications giving an imbalance of the imprinted genes occur at higher incidence due to ART. This is interesting as ART mothers are typically older so an increased incidence of uniparental disomy could be expected.

It is difficult to know whether the abnormal methylation causing these imprinting defects is as a result of one of the many processes encompassed by ART or associated with subfertility. Studies of superovulated oocytes from infertile women have shown altered methylation (Sato et al., 2007).

Genomic imprinting may be less complete when immature gametes are used (Tesarik & Mendoza, 1996). There is currently no evidence of increased numbers of individuals with imprinting defects conceived by PESA and TESA but numbers are too small to draw any firm conclusions and further study is required.

Two particular imprinting syndromes which seem to be at higher rates following ART are Angelman syndrome and Beckwith Weidemann syndrome (BWS).

BWS is an overgrowth syndrome where individuals are affected by neonatal hypoglycaemia, macroglossia, macrosomia and midline abdominal wall defects (omphalocele, umbilical hernia, diastasis recti). It is caused by uniparental disomy or imprinting defect affecting chromosome 11p15 (Shuman et al., 2005). Several studies have found increased rates of BWS in children born following ART (Halliday et al., 2004; Maher et al., 2003). Studies in the UK, USA and France have found children with BWS were more likely to have been conceived by ART (Chang et al., 2005; Gicquel et al., 2003; Maher et al., 2003). These cases were largely caused by imprinting defects. One case report describes a family where two children have been born with BWS, one following IVF and one spontaneously conceived (following years of infertility treatment) suggesting in this case the IVF was not the cause (Strawn et al., 2010). Interestingly in animals conceived by IVF or nuclear transfer a large offspring syndrome has been described which shares similarities with BWS (Gicquel et al., 2003).

Angelman syndrome affects âĹij1 in 16 000 children and is characterized by severe intellectual disability, speech impairment, a happy demeanour, ataxia, seizures and microcephaly. It is caused by abnormalities affecting the maternal copy of chromosome 15q11-13. Overall 5% of cases are associated with an imprinting defect. Early case reports described cases of Angelman syndrome conceived using ICSI with AS secondary to loss of methylation. A higher proportion of cases of AS in children born using ART seem to be as a result of methylation defects. Interestingly a German cohort found an excess of AS cases again with methylation defects in children spontaneously conceived by subfertile couples (Lidegaard et al., 2005).

Two case reports have described hypomethylation of the paternally derived H19/IGF2 locus in infants with Russell-Silver syndrome conceived by ICSI (Chopra et al., 2010; Douzgou et al., 2008). Several other children born following ART with this syndrome have also been described. Beyond the classically recognised imprinting syndromes, decreased methylation has been found in spontaneously conceived individuals with neural tube defects (Wang et al. 2010). Further work is needed to see if this is consistent with the explanation for the possible increase in ART.

Many of the imprinting syndromes are very rare. Even if ART increases the risk of these disorders by two or three times it will still be very difficult to detect this increased risk. The

Danish National IVF cohort study found no cases of imprinting disorders in the 6052 children born following IVF between 1995 and 2001 (Lidegaard et al., 2005).

6. Association of malformations with different types of ART

Most studies have found few differences in the malformation rates between different types of ART. It could be hypothesized that the more invasive techniques are likely to carry a higher risk of malformation but many techniques have not yet been used enough to show definitive results. It seems likely that techniques allowing in vivo fertilization (eg GIFT) are safer than those relying on in vitro fertilization. To support this no increase in malformations have been observed following ovarian stimulation (**?**).

An early study of 91 infants born following embryo cryopreservation found a relative risk of a major malformation of 1.4 including cases of Beckwith Weidemann syndrome and Downs syndrome (Sutcliffe et al., 1995). More recent work has shown an increase in aneuploidys in embryos following cryopreservation (Guran et al., 2010). Other work has shown no increase in malformations when using frozen embryos over fresh (Li et al., 2010). A systematic review found comparable results for IVF using fresh or frozen embryos (Wennerholm et al., 2009).

Some of the most definitive work shows that children conceived by ART are at a higher risk of reproductive tract anomalies, particularly hypospadius in boys conceived by ICSI (Funke et al., 2010; Klln et al., 2005b; **?**). Prematurity, low birthweight, and multiple gestation, are indirect risk factors for developing male genital malformations but in infants with normal birthweight or from singleton pregnancies, ICSI is a specific risk factor for hypospadias.(Funke et al., 2010) More boys conceived by ICSI were also found to have undescended testes requiring surgery (Ludwig, Katalinic, Thyen, Sutcliffe, Diedrich & Ludwig, 2009). In ICSI the sperm has been unable to fertilise the egg and is therefore in some way abnormal. It is possible that men who are only able to have children by ICSI, in some cases pass on this defect to their sons. In ICSI using epididimal or testicular sperm (MESA and TESA) a systematic review (Woldringh et al., 2010) found there is not enough data to reliably say if this affects the rate of congenital malformations in subsequent offspring although one study had found a higher rate of polyploidy in abortuses (Mateu et al., 2010).

Early reports from cases series of individuals conceived following preimplantation genetic diagnosis show no risk of malformations over ICSI but there was an increased perinatal death rate (Liebaers et al., 2010).

7. Conclusions

There is mounting evidence that infants conceived by these methods are at slightly higher risk of congenital abnormalities overall with particularly compelling evidence for imprinting syndromes and urogenital malformations. Some of the increased risk of congenital malformations following ART appears to be the effect of subfertility rather than ART per se.

This conclusion is echoed by a recent ESHRE position statement which states "Children from couples who get pregnant after assisted reproduction techniques, like IVF/ICSI, have a 40-50% increased risk for a birth defect. A similar increased risk has been reported for subfertile couples who get pregnant spontaneously after a prolonged time period. This increased risk seems thus mainly be due to parental characteristics from the infertility status and not to the treatment given."

It is still early days. Louise Brown, the first person born by IVF is now in her 30s and has given birth to a spontaneously conceived child. The oldest person born by ICSI is only 20. There are case reports of people born following ART with a range of syndromes for example Goldenhar syndrome and Rubinstein-Taybi syndrome conceived by ICSI (Balci et al., 2008). It is too early to say if this is a chance finding or a genuine association. As the number of people born following ART increases and they move through their lives It is important they continue to be monitored particularly as new techniques are developed so people using these techniques, which overall are relatively safe, can be given an accurate picture of the risks they face and future children can be monitored appropriately.

8. References

Al-Fifi, S., Al-Binali, A., Al-Shahrani, M., Shafiq, H., Bahar, M., Almushait, M., Sobandi, L. & Eskandar, M. (2009). Congenital anomalies and other perinatal outcomes in ICSI vs. naturally conceived pregnancies: a comparative study., *Journal of assisted reproduction and genetics* 26(7): 377–81.

Amor, D. J. & Halliday, J. (2008). A review of known imprinting syndromes and their association with assisted reproduction technologies., *Human reproduction (Oxford, England)* 23(12): 2826–34.

Australian in vitro fertilisation collaborative group (1985). High incidence of preterm births and early losses in pregnancy after in vitro fertilisation., *British medical journal (Clinical research ed.)* 291(6503): 1160–3.

Bahtiyar, M. O., Campbell, K., Dulay, A. T., Kontic-Vucinic, O., Weeks, B. P., Friedman, A. H. & Copel, J. A. (2010). Is the rate of congenital heart defects detected by fetal echocardiography among pregnancies conceived by in vitro fertilization really increased?: a case-historical control study., *Journal of ultrasound in medicine : official journal of the American Institute of Ultrasound in Medicine* 29(6): 917–22.

Balci, S., Engiz, O., Alikasifoglu, M., Esinler, I. & Sinan Beksac, M. (2008). Association of assisted reproductive technology with twinning and congenital anomalies., *Indian journal of pediatrics* 75(6): 638–40.

Bettio, D., Venci, A. & Levi Setti, P. E. (2008). Chromosomal abnormalities in miscarriages after different assisted reproduction procedures., *Placenta* 29 Suppl B: 126–8.

Bofinger, M., NEEDHAM, D., Saldana, L., Sosnowski, J. & Blough, R. (1999). 45, X/46, x, r (y) karyotype transmitted by father to son after intracytoplasmic sperm injection for oligospermia: a case report, *Journal of reproductive medicine* 44(7): 645–648.

Chang, A. S., Moley, K. H., Wangler, M., Feinberg, A. P. & Debaun, M. R. (2005). Association between Beckwith-Wiedemann syndrome and assisted reproductive technology: a case series of 19 patients., *Fertility and sterility* 83(2): 349–54.

Chopra, M., Amor, D. J., Sutton, L., Algar, E. & Mowat, D. (2010). Russell-Silver syndrome due to paternal H19/IGF2 hypomethylation in a patient conceived using intracytoplasmic sperm injection., *Reproductive biomedicine online* 20(6): 843–7.

Douzgou, S., Mingarelli, R., Tarani, L., De Crescenzo, A. & Riccio, A. (2008). Silver-Russell syndrome following in vitro fertilization., *Pediatric and developmental pathology : the official journal of the Society for Pediatric Pathology and the Paediatric Pathology Society* 11(4): 329–31.

Ericson, A. & Källén, B. (2001). Congenital malformations in infants born after IVF: a population-based study., *Human reproduction (Oxford, England)* 16(3): 504–9.

Foresta, C. & Ferlin, A. (2001). Offspring conceived by intracytoplasmic sperm injection, *Lancet* 358(9289): 1270.

Funke, S., Flach, E., Kiss, I., Sándor, J., Vida, G., Bódis, J. & Ertl, T. (2010). Male reproductive tract abnormalities: more common after assisted reproduction?, *Early human development* 86(9): 547–50.

Gallati, S., Hess, S., Galié-Wunder, D., Berger-Menz, E. & Böhlen, D. (2009). Cystic fibrosis transmembrane conductance regulator mutations in azoospermic and oligospermic men and their partners., *Reproductive biomedicine online* 19(5): 685–94.

Gicquel, C., Gaston, V., Mandelbaum, J., Siffroi, J., Flahault, A. & Le Bouc, Y. (2003). In vitro fertilization may increase the risk of Beckwith-Wiedemann syndrome related to the abnormal imprinting of the kcnq1ot gene, *American journal of human genetics* 72(5): 1338.

Guran, S., Rosti, R. O., Sarici, S. m., Torun, D., Kozan, S. & Bahçe, M. (2010). Rare chromosomal complement of trisomy 21 in a boy conceived only by IVF., *Reproductive biomedicine online* 21(5): 721–2; author reply 723.

Halliday, J. L., Ukoumunne, O. C., Baker, H. W. G., Breheny, S., Jaques, A. M., Garrett, C., Healy, D. & Amor, D. (2010). Increased risk of blastogenesis birth defects, arising in the first 4 weeks of pregnancy, after assisted reproductive technologies., *Human reproduction (Oxford, England)* 25(1): 59–65.

Halliday, J., Oke, K., Breheny, S., Algar, E. & J Amor, D. (2004). Beckwith-Wiedemann syndrome and IVF: a case-control study., *American journal of human genetics* 75(3): 526–8.

Hansen, M., Bower, C., Milne, E., de Klerk, N. & Kurinczuk, J. J. (2005). Assisted reproductive technologies and the risk of birth defects–a systematic review., *Human reproduction (Oxford, England)* 20(2): 328–38.

Hansen, M., Kurinczuk, J. J., Bower, C. & Webb, S. (2002). The risk of major birth defects after intracytoplasmic sperm injection and in vitro fertilization., *The New England journal of medicine* 346(10): 725–30.

Helmerhorst, F., Perquin, D., Donker, D. & Keirse, M. (2004). Perinatal outcome of singletons and twins after assisted conception: a systematic review of controlled studies, *BMJ* 328(7434): 261.

Holmes, L. B. (1976). Current concepts in genetics. congenital malformations., *The New England journal of medicine* 295(4): 204–7.

Human Fertilisation and Embryology Authority (2011). Fertility facts and figures, *Human reproduction* pp. 21–4.

Hvidtjørn, D., Grove, J., Schendel, D., Svaerke, C., Schieve, L., Uldall, P., Ernst, E., Jacobsson, B. & Thorsen, P. (2010). Multiplicity and early gestational age contribute to an increased risk of cerebral palsy from assisted conception: a population-based cohort study, *Human reproduction (Oxford, England)* 25(8): 2115–23.

Hvidtjørn, D., Grove, J., Schendel, D., Vaeth, M., Ernst, E., Nielsen, L. & Thorsen, P. (2006). Cerebral palsy among children born after in vitro fertilization: the role of preterm delivery–a population-based, cohort study, *Pediatrics* 118(2): 475–82.

ICMART (2008). Presentation of preliminary data for 2004, *Human reproduction (Oxford, England)* .

Jackson, R., Gibson, K., Wu, Y. & Croughan, M. (2004). Perinatal outcomes in singletons following in vitro fertilization: a meta-analysis, *Obstetrics & Gynecology* 103(3): 551.

Källén, B., Finnström, O., Nygren, K. & Olausson, P. (2005a). In vitro fertilization (IVF) in Sweden: infant outcome after different IVF fertilization methods, *Fertility and sterility* 84(3): 611–7.

Klln, B., Finnstrm, O., Nygren, K. & Olausson, P. (2005b). In vitro fertilization (IVF) in Sweden: risk for congenital malformations after different IVF methods, *Birth Defects Research Part A: Clinical and Molecular Teratology* 73(3): 162–169.

Källén, B., Olausson, P. & Nygren, K. (2002). Neonatal outcome in pregnancies from ovarian stimulation, *Obstetrics & Gynecology* 100(3): 414.

Koşar, P. A., Ozçelik, N. & Koşar, A. (2010). Cytogenetic abnormalities detected in patients with non-obstructive azoospermia and severe oligozoospermia., *Journal of assisted reproduction and genetics* 27(1): 17–21.

Lancaster, P. A. (1987). Congenital malformations after in-vitro fertilisation., *Lancet* 2(8572): 1392–3.

Li, H., Qiao, J., Chi, H., Chen, X., Liu, P. & Ma, C. (2010). Comparison of the major malformation rate of children conceived from cryopreserved embryos and fresh embryos, *Chinese medical journal* 123(14): 1893–7.

Lidegaard, O., Pinborg, A. & Andersen, A. (2005). Imprinting diseases and IVF: Danish National IVF cohort study, *Human reproduction (Oxford, England)* 20(4): 950–4.

Lie, R. T., Lyngstadaas, A., Ørstavik, K. H., Bakketeig, L. S., Jacobsen, G. & Tanbo, T. (2005). Birth defects in children conceived by ICSI compared with children conceived by other IVF-methods; a meta-analysis., *International journal of epidemiology* 34(3): 696–701.

Liebaers, I., Desmyttere, S., Verpoest, W., De Rycke, M., Staessen, C., Sermon, K., Devroey, P., Haentjens, P. & Bonduelle, M. (2010). Report on a consecutive series of 581 children born after blastomere biopsy for preimplantation genetic diagnosis., *Human reproduction (Oxford, England)* 25(1): 275–82.

Ludwig, A. K., Katalinic, A., Thyen, U., Sutcliffe, A. G., Diedrich, K. & Ludwig, M. (2009). Physical health at 5.5 years of age of term-born singletons after intracytoplasmic sperm injection: results of a prospective, controlled, single-blinded study., *Fertility and sterility* 91(1): 115–24.

Ludwig, A., Katalinic, A., Entenmann, A., Thyen, U., Sutcliffe, A., Diedrich, K. & Ludwig, M. (2009). Can we sense ART? The blinded examiner is not blind–a problem with follow-up studies on children born after assisted reproduction, *Fertility and sterility* 92(3): 950–952.

Maher, E. R., Brueton, L. A., Bowdin, S. C., Luharia, A., Cooper, W., Cole, T. R., Macdonald, F., Sampson, J. R., Barratt, C. L., Reik, W. & Hawkins, M. M. (2003). Beckwith-Wiedemann syndrome and assisted reproduction technology (ART)., *Journal of medical genetics* 40(1): 62–4.

Mateu, E., Rodrigo, L., Martínez, M. C., Peinado, V., Milán, M., Gil-Salom, M., Martínez-Jabaloyas, J. M., Remohí, J., Pellicer, A. & Rubio, C. (2010). Aneuploidies in embryos and spermatozoa from patients with Y chromosome microdeletions., *Fertility and sterility* 94(7): 2874–7.

MRC Working Party on Children Conceived by In Vitro Fertilisation (1990). Births in Great Britain resulting from assisted conception, 1978-87., *BMJ (Clinical research ed.)* 300(6734): 1229–33.

Odom, L. N. & Segars, J. (2010). Imprinting disorders and assisted reproductive technology., *Current opinion in endocrinology, diabetes, and obesity* 17(6): 517–22.

Palermo, G., Joris, H., Devroey, P. & Van Steirteghem, A. (1992). Pregnancies after intracytoplasmic injection of single spermatozoon into an oocyte, *The Lancet* 340(8810): 17–18.

Reefhuis, J., Honein, M. A., Schieve, L. A., Correa, A., Hobbs, C. A., Rasmussen, S. A. & National Birth Defects Prevention Study (2009). Assisted reproductive technology and major structural birth defects in the United States., *Human reproduction (Oxford, England)* 24(2): 360–6.

Rimm, A. A., Katayama, A. C., Diaz, M. & Katayama, K. P. (2004). A meta-analysis of controlled studies comparing major malformation rates in IVF and ICSI infants with naturally conceived children., *Journal of assisted reproduction and genetics* 21(12): 437–43.

Rimm, A. A., Katayama, A. C. & Katayama, K. P. (2011). A meta-analysis of the impact of IVF and ICSI on major malformations after adjusting for the effect of subfertility., *Journal of assisted reproduction and genetics* .

Rubio, C. (2010). Update on preimplantation genetic diagnosis for chromosomal abnormalities., *Expert review of molecular diagnostics* 10(8): 973–6.

Sato, A., Otsu, E., Negishi, H., Utsunomiya, T. & Arima, T. (2007). Aberrant DNA methylation of imprinted loci in superovulated oocytes., *Human reproduction (Oxford, England)* 22(1): 26–35.

Schieve, L., Cohen, B., Nannini, A., Ferre, C., Reynolds, M., Zhang, Z., Jeng, G., Macaluso, M. & Wright, V. (2007). A population-based study of maternal and perinatal outcomes associated with assisted reproductive technology in Massachusetts, *Maternal and child health journal* 11(6): 517–525.

Schieve, L., Meikle, S., Ferre, C., Peterson, H., Jeng, G. & Wilcox, L. (2002). Low and very low birth weight in infants conceived with use of assisted reproductive technology, *New England Journal of Medicine* 346(10): 731–737.

Shuman, C., Smith, A. & Weksberg, R. (2005). Beckwith-Wiedemann syndrome, *GeneReviews at GeneTests: Medical Genetics Information Resource (database online). Seattle: University of Washington* .

Simpson, J. L. (1996). Registration of congenital anomalies in ART populations: pitfalls., *Human reproduction (Oxford, England)* 11 Suppl 4: 81–8.

Spinner, N. B., Saitta, S. C., Delaney, D. P., Colliton, R., Zderic, S. A., Ruchelli, E., Zackai, E. & Kolon, T. F. (2008). Intracytoplasmic sperm injection (ICSI) with transmission of a ring(Y) chromosome and ovotesticular disorder of sex development in offspring., *American journal of medical genetics. Part A* 146A(14): 1828–31.

Stark, Z., Storen, R., Bennetts, B., Savarirayan, R. & Jamieson, R. V. (2011). Isolated hypogonadotropic hypogonadism with SOX2 mutation and anophthalmia/microphthalmia in offspring., *European journal of human genetics : EJHG* .

Strawn, E. Y., Bick, D. & Swanson, A. (2010). Is it the patient or the IVF? Beckwith-Wiedemann syndrome in both spontaneous and assisted reproductive conceptions., *Fertility and sterility* 94(2): 754.e1–2.

Strömberg, B., Dahlquist, G., Ericson, A., Finnström, O., Köster, M. & Stjernqvist, K. (2002). Neurological sequelae in children born after in-vitro fertilisation: a population-based study, *Lancet* 359(9305): 461–5.

Sutcliffe, A., D'souza, S., Cadman, J., Richards, B., McKinlay, I. & Lieberman, B. (1995). Minor congenital anomalies, major congenital malformations and development in children conceived from cryopreserved embryos, *Human Reproduction* 10(12): 3332.

Tararbit, K., Houyel, L., Bonnet, D., De Vigan, C., Lelong, N., Goffinet, F. & Khoshnood, B. (2011). Risk of congenital heart defects associated with assisted reproductive technologies: a population-based evaluation., *European heart journal* 32(4): 500–8.

Tesarik, J. & Mendoza, C. (1996). Genomic imprinting abnormalities: a new potential risk of assisted reproduction., *Molecular human reproduction* 2(5): 295–8.

Turan, N., Katari, S., Gerson, L., Chalian, R., Foster, M., Gaughan, J., Coutifaris, C. & Sapienza, C. (2010). Inter- and intra-individual variation in allele-specific DNA methylation and gene expression in children conceived using assisted reproductive technology, *PLoS genetics* 6(7).

Vicdan, A., Vicdan, K., Günalp, S., Kence, A., Akarsu, C., Işik, A. Z. & Sözen, E. (2004). Genetic aspects of human male infertility: the frequency of chromosomal abnormalities and Y chromosome microdeletions in severe male factor infertility., *European journal of obstetrics, gynecology, and reproductive biology* 117(1): 49–54.

Wen, S. W., Leader, A., White, R. R., Léveillé, M.-C., Wilkie, V., Zhou, J. & Walker, M. C. (2010). A comprehensive assessment of outcomes in pregnancies conceived by in vitro fertilization/intracytoplasmic sperm injection., *European journal of obstetrics, gynecology, and reproductive biology* 150(2): 160–5.

Wennerholm, U., Söderström-Anttila, V., Bergh, C., Aittomäki, K., Hazekamp, J., Nygren, K., Selbing, A. & Loft, A. (2009). Children born after cryopreservation of embryos or oocytes: a systematic review of outcome data, *Human Reproduction* 24(9): 2158.

Woldringh, G. H., Besselink, D. E., Tillema, A. H. J., Hendriks, J. C. M. & Kremer, J. A. M. (2010). Karyotyping, congenital anomalies and follow-up of children after intracytoplasmic sperm injection with non-ejaculated sperm: a systematic review., *Human reproduction update* 16(1): 12–9.

Zhu, J., Hvidtjørn, D., Basso, O., Obel, C., Thorsen, P., Uldall, P. & Olsen, J. (2010). Parental infertility and cerebral palsy in children, *Human reproduction (Oxford, England)* 25(12): 3142–5.

Zhu, J. L., Basso, O., Obel, C., Bille, C. & Olsen, J. (2006). Infertility, infertility treatment, and congenital malformations: Danish national birth cohort., *BMJ (Clinical research ed.)* 333(7570): 679.